DIABETES

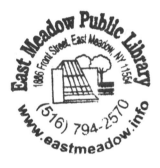

LICENSE, DISCLAIMER OF LIABILITY, AND LIMITED WARRANTY

DIABETES

Dr. Nicola Cowap
Nicola M. Parry

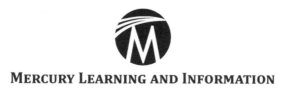

MERCURY LEARNING AND INFORMATION

Dulles, Virginia
Boston, Massachusetts
New Delhi

Publisher: David Pallai
MERCURY LEARNING AND INFORMATION
22841 Quicksilver Drive
Dulles, VA 20166
info@merclearning.com
www.merclearning.com
(800) 232-0223

This book is printed on acid-free paper.

Dr. Nicola Cowap and Nicola M. Parry. *Diabetes.*
ISBN: 978-1-938549-18-2

Library of Congress Control Number: 2014950123
1516 17 3 2 1   Printed in the United States of America

Our titles are available for adoption, license, or bulk purchase by institutions,
corporations, etc.   ·
For additional information, please contact the Customer Service Dept. at
(800)232-0223(toll free).

Contents

Management of Diabetes

Monitoring Blood Sugar, Including the Use of
a Blood Sugar Meter and HbA1c Testing

Pills to Help Control Blood Sugar Levels,
Including Metformin, Sulfonylurea Drugs,
and Others

Insulin Therapy

PART SIX

Keys to Living with Diabetes

CHAPTER 16

Stopping Smoking

CHAPTER 17

Diet, Nutrition, and Management of Obesity

CHAPTER 18

Physical Activity

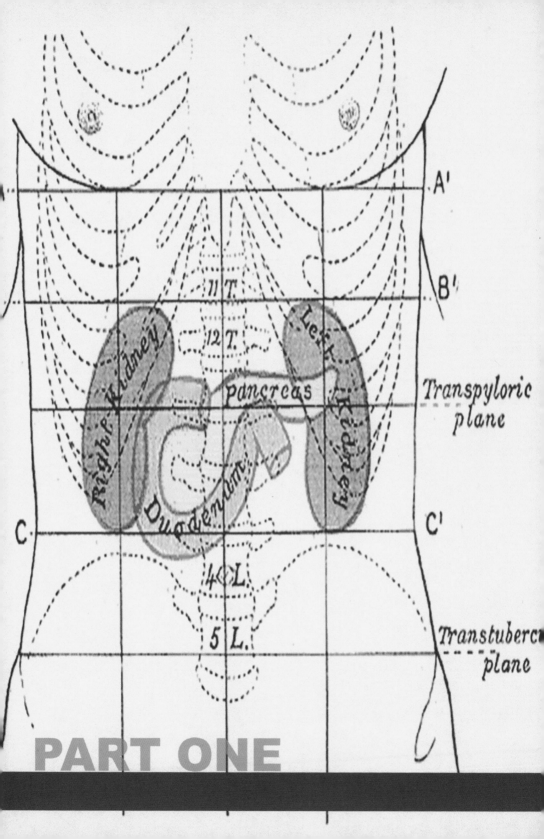

A'

B'

11 T.

12 T.

Right Kidney

pancreas

Left Kidney

Duodenum

Transpyloric
plane

C

C'

4 L.

5 L.

Transtuberc...
plane

PART ONE

Diabetes Basics

In Part One, we will discuss the basic definitions of prediabetes and diabetes. We will answer questions about blood sugar and the pancreas, and then expand our discussion to how the pancreas works to control blood sugar levels. Finally, we take a look at how the pancreas relates to diabetes, and what happens when it stops working.

CHAPTER 1
Introduction to Diabetes

CHAPTER 2
The Pancreas

CHAPTER 3
Normal Pancreatic Function

Introduction to Diabetes

1. What is diabetes?

The term **diabetes** comes from the full name of the condition known medically as **diabetes mellitus**: *diabetes* comes from a Greek word meaning "to siphon," and *mellitus* comes from a Latin word meaning "sweet." This is because diabetes involves a build up of abnormally high levels of **sugar** in the blood because it cannot leave the blood and travel into **cells** where it is needed for **energy**. As a result, it passes out through the kidneys into the urine. This happens if the body does not produce enough **insulin**, or if it cannot use insulin properly. In both these cases, the body is no longer able to control blood sugar levels, so the sugar remains in the bloodstream.

> **DEFINITION**
> **Diabetes** is a condition where the body cannot process sugar in the diet into energy.

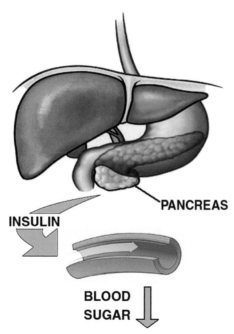

INSULIN

PANCREAS

BLOOD SUGAR

▲ **FIGURE 1.1**
Insulin from the Pancreas Allows Blood Sugar to Move into Cells for Energy.

See how insulin works to control blood sugar levels normally, and in diabetes:

http://blausen.com/?Topic=7010

ON THE WEB

If left untreated or poorly controlled, diabetes can lead to serious health problems. It is the fastest growing disease in the world, and the seventh leading cause of death in the United States.

2. What is prediabetes?

Prediabetes is when your blood sugar levels are higher than normal, but not high enough to be classified as diabetes.

DEFINITION

In the United States, the prevalence of prediabetes is increasing. About one-third of people aged 20 years and older have prediabetes, but only about 11% are aware of it, because most people do not have symptoms.

To determine if you have prediabetes, visit:

http://www.youtube.com/watch?v=WRI-vEjNvyA

ON THE WEB

Even though the levels of glucose in prediabetes are not as high as in full-blown diabetes, the long-term damage due to excess blood sugar begins to set in even at this early stage of prediabetes, especially in the heart and circulatory system. People with prediabetes therefore have a higher risk of developing type 2 diabetes, as well as the serious health problems that can go along with

For more information about other risk factors that can raise your risk of developing prediabetes, visit:

http://www.cdc.gov/diabetes/consumer/prediabetes.htm

ON THE WEB

it, including heart disease and stroke. Your doctor may test you for prediabetes, especially if you are overweight and over 45 years of age, because age and excessive weight can be risk factors for the condition.

The body mass index (BMI) is a way to tell whether you are a healthy weight for your height. Although this measurement doesn't directly measure your body fat, it is still the recommended way to determine whether you are overweight or obese.

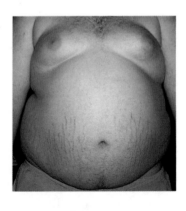

▶ FIGURE 1.2
Being Overweight or Obese Puts You at Risk for Prediabetes.

SOURCE: Wikimedia

The BMI is a calculation of weight relative to height, and will place you in one of 4 categories:

Table 1.1 BMI categories for adults

WEIGHT STATUS	BMI
Underweight	Less than 18.5
Normal	18.5 – 24.9
Overweight	25 – 29.9
Obese	30.0 or more

SOURCE: Based on the Centers for Disease Control and Prevention's, "How is BMI calculated and interpreted?", http://www.cdc.gov/healthyweight/assessing/bmi/adult_bmi/index.html

The risk of developing prediabetes begins to increase at a BMI of 25, and the risk is about 5 times higher in obese people with a BMI of 30 or more.

However, having prediabetes doesn't automatically mean you will definitely develop type 2 diabetes. It can even be considered a wake-up call and a good opportunity to get healthy, because at this stage, there is still time to turn things around by making appropriate lifestyle changes to prevent the development of diabetes and the long-term serious health effects that go along with it.

To calculate your BMI, visit:

http://www.nhlbi.nih.gov/guidelines/obesity/BMI/bmicalc.htm

If you have prediabetes, regardless of your starting weight, lowering your BMI by just five points can significantly reduce your risk of developing diabetes. This can be accomplished by a three-part approach that involves keeping a healthy weight, eating a healthy diet, and exercising daily, all of which can help get your blood sugar level back to normal again.

If you are overweight, the most important goal is to lose weight, and keeping a healthy diet is essential to achieve this. Reducing portion size and making better food choices are key factors here. For example, you should reduce how much fat you eat with each meal, choose more vegetables and fruit, eat

To learn more about recommendations for management of obesity, see Document 1.1.ObesManage.

http://www.racgp.org.au/afp/2013/august/obesity/

less meat, and choose fish, chicken, and lean cuts of beef for protein. If necessary, seek the help of a Registered Dietitian to find out how much food, and what types, you should be eating.

Regular exercise is another important part of the approach to reducing your BMI. Exercise helps your body to use insulin from the pancreas to convert food into energy, keeping your blood sugar levels lower. Introducing moderate-intensity physical activity into your life, such as just walking for 30 minutes daily, can be highly effective for people, especially if you are not currently exercising regularly. But be sure to seek advice from your physician before starting any new exercise regime.

For more information about healthy habits that can help reduce your risk of developing type 2 diabetes, visit:

http://www.cdc.gov/diabetes/prevention/about.htm

Prediabetes therefore represents a high-risk state for the development of diabetes. If people with prediabetes do not make healthy lifestyle changes, up to 30% will develop full-blown diabetes within 5 years, and even more will develop it over the longer term.

3. Why is high blood sugar a problem?

High blood sugar levels (medically known as hyperglycemia) from uncontrolled diabetes can lead to serious health problems. In the short term, for example, ketoacidosis, or diabetic coma, can occur. In the longer term, high blood sugar levels can damage different parts of the body. Diabetes is a leading cause of kidney disease, new cases of blindness, and lower limb amputation. It also raises your risk of heart disease and stroke.

4. Can diabetes be cured?

For results of the study showing how weight loss surgery can result in diabetes remission, visit:

http://www.webmd.com/diet/weight-loss-surgery/news/20130919/weight-loss-surgery-can-improve-long-term-diabetes-control-study-says

Type 2 diabetes cannot be cured, but if it is managed properly, patients with diabetes can live long, happy lives.

There is evidence to suggest that if patients with type 2 diabetes undergo weight loss surgery (also known as bariatric surgery) within 5 years of being diagnosed, their disease can go into long-term remission that lasts longer than 5 years.

The two most common types of weight loss surgery are gastric banding and gastric bypass. They work by reducing the amount of food the stomach can hold, and reducing food absorption by the stomach and small intestine. After both types of surgery, patients eat less and feel full quickly after eating small meals. This is because the surgery shrinks the stomach from the size of a football to about the size of a golf ball that can only hold about a half-cup of food.

 For additional information about the effect of weight loss surgery on causing diabetes remission, see Document 1.2.RemissionWt.

http://www.ncbi.nlm.nih.gov/pmc/articles/PMC3801373/

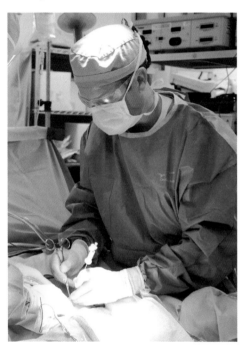

The Pancreas

5. What is the pancreas?

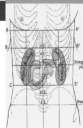

The pancreas is a V-shaped gland in the upper part of the abdomen, located on the left side of the body, and is about six inches long. It lies behind the stomach and has a connection to the duodenum (the first section of the intestine, which is connected to the stomach) via a tube known as a duct.

Ductal Anatomy of Liver and Pancreas

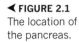

◄ FIGURE 2.1
The location of the pancreas.

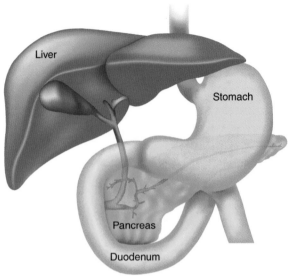

Liver

Stomach

Pancreas

Duodenum

SOURCE: Illustration adapted from www.aokainc.com

It is an important gland with two main functions: digestion and blood sugar control. The pancreas makes special proteins known as enzymes that help us digest food, and these enzymes drain from the gland to the intestine in the duct. It also makes hormones that are important in controlling our blood sugar. In particular, it continually releases just enough of one hormone, insulin, to keep blood sugar levels under control constantly throughout the day. It is when the pancreas fails in this function of blood sugar control that diabetes develops.

To learn more about the function of the pancreas, visit:

http://www.youtube.com/watch?v=NZ4zcrTzUjA

ON THE WEB

6. What is sugar?

Sugar comes from the breakdown of dietary carbohydrates in substances like fruits, vegetables, grains, and milk. With the help of the pancreas, the body digests these substances soon after they are eaten, and changes them into sugar, which enters the bloodstream and travels to the different cells in the body to act as fuel to help them function.

Sugar, or glucose, is a naturally occurring nutrient that makes foods taste sweet. It is a simple carbohydrate, and is the main energy source for most cells in the body.

ON THE WEB

The cells of the body work best when they are supplied with just enough sugar to provide them with energy. While all cells need energy, most of them can use fats as an alternate energy source. Nerve cells and red blood cells, however, cannot use fats for energy—they can only use sugar as an energy supply. So regulation of blood sugar levels is especially important to keep the nervous system functioning properly, for example.

To learn more about carbohydrates and sugar, visit:

http://www.youtube.com/watch?v=Tg4j5yC9QpU

7. What are the components of the pancreas, and what do they do?

Although physically the pancreas is a single gland organ, it functions as two different types of gland in one: an exocrine gland and an endocrine gland. Both gland types work together to help digest meals (exocrine gland) and to send signals to other regions of the body where nutrients are being processed and are traveling to the cells of the body (endocrine gland).

The exocrine gland component makes up about 99% of the pancreas, and plays a vital role in the digestion of food, producing enzymes that are critical to help digest carbohydrates, fats, and proteins in the diet. It releases these enzymes into pancreatic juice, which is delivered into the duodenum via the duct, to help breakdown food as it leaves the stomach. These enzymes include: amylase, to break down carbohydrates like starch into more simple sugars like glucose; lipase, to break down larger and more complex fats like triglycerides into smaller fatty acid components; and trypsin and chymotrypsin, enzymes that break down protein substances into their smaller amino acid components.

The endocrine gland component makes up the remaining 1% of the gland, and is composed of many islets of Langerhans. These are small clusters of cells, also known as islet cells, which produce hormones important for control of blood sugar levels.

For more information about carbohydrates, fats, and proteins, visit:

http://www.nlm.nih.gov/medlineplus/carbohydrates.html

http://www.nlm.nih.gov/medlineplus/dietaryfats.html

http://www.nlm.nih.gov/medlineplus/ency/article/002467.htm

In a healthy adult person, there are about 1 million islets in the pancreas. In patients with diabetes, the islets do not function adequately, and there are also fewer of them.

PRACTICAL TIP

In the islets, there are numerous types of cells that produce different hormones. The islets also have a rich blood supply, allowing easy access to the bloodstream for these hormones.

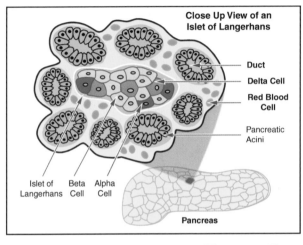

Close Up View of an
Islet of Langerhans

Duct

Delta Cell

Red Blood
Cell

Pancreatic
Acini

Islet of   Beta   Alpha
Langerhans Cell   Cell

Pancreas

◀ FIGURE 2.2
An islet surrounded by exocrine gland cells in the pancreas.

SOURCE: Illustration adapted from www.homebusiness andfamilylife.com

To learn more about the endocrine function of the pancreas, visit:

http://www.youtube.com/watch?v=4VszMzQ2tmE

ON THE WEB

Three cell types predominate in the islets: **alpha cells** make up about 15% of the hormone-producing cells, and these produce **glucagon**, a hormone that increases blood sugar levels. **Beta cells** are located in the center of the islets and make up about 75% of the cells. They produce insulin, a hormone that works to lower blood sugar levels. Another hormone, **somatostatin**, is produced by **delta cells**, which account for about 5% of the islet cells. It has numerous functions, one of which is to help regulate the release of insulin and glucagon.

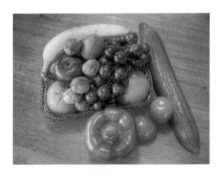

Normal Pancreatic Function

8. How does insulin control blood sugar?

Insulin and glucagon are the two main hormones produced by the pancreas, and they are critical for the regulation of blood sugar levels.

The pancreas carefully senses how much sugar is present in the blood. If the levels are too high, the pancreas releases insulin into the blood so it can help sugar move into cells that need it as an energy source to function properly. This in turn lowers the levels in the blood.

ON THE WEB

To learn more about the function of insulin, visit:

http://www.youtube.com/watch?v=IrotOPgSkR4

On the contrary, if levels are too low, the pancreas releases glucagon instead. This causes cells in the liver to release sugar into the blood, thereby increasing the levels in the blood again. And when blood sugar levels increase again, the pancreas stops releasing glucagon, and once again switches to release insulin, and so forth. This is how the pancreas helps keep your sugar levels steady in response to eating. During a meal, when your blood sugar starts to rise, it releases insulin to lower sugar levels. And in between meals, when sugar levels drop again, the pancreas releases glucagon to increase it back to normal.

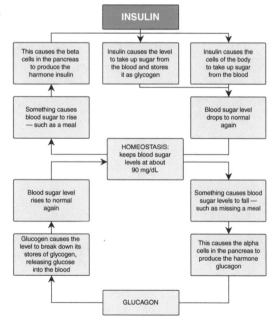

INSULIN

This causes the beta cells in the pancreas to produce the harmone insulin

Insulin causes the level to take up sugar from the blood and stores it as glycogen

Insulin causes the cells of the body to take up sugar from the blood

Something causes blood sugar to rise — such as a meal

Blood sugar level drops to normal again

HOMEOSTASIS: keeps blood sugar levels at about 90 mg/dL

Blood sugar level rises to normal again

Something causes blood sugar levels to fall — such as missing a meal

Glucogen causes the level to break down its stores of glycogen, releasing glucose into the blood

This causes the alpha cells in the pancreas to produce the harmone glucagon

GLUCAGON

▲ FIGURE 3.1

How the hormones of the pancreas regulate blood sugar.

SOURCE: Illustration adapted from www.lamission.edu

9. What should my blood sugar level be?

When you eat a meal, blood sugar levels will increase, and in a person without diabetes, the levels usually don't rise above 140 mg/dL because the pancreas regulates it tightly. This keeps sugar levels in the blood within a narrow range throughout different times of the day. A normal fasting blood sugar level (the level when you have not eaten for at least 8 hours) for someone without diabetes is 70–100 mg/dL. And one or two hours after a meal, blood sugar levels are below 100 mg/dL in most people without diabetes.

For more information about recommended blood sugar goals, visit:

http://www.nlm.nih.gov/medlineplus/ency/patientinstructions/000086.htm

But in people with diabetes, the pancreas doesn't function effectively. Insulin release is defective, and these patients therefore cannot control their blood sugar levels adequately.

If levels increase above 180–200 mg/dL, this prevents the kidneys being able to stop sugar being lost as they filter blood passing through them. In these instances, sugar therefore spills out into the urine. When levels become even higher, around 400 mg/dL and above, this is when it is possible to see changes in mental function.

To learn more about hyperglycemia, visit:

http://www.youtube.com/watch?v=rz75JK1Z_z0&list=TLuOlF4EK6iPW0WoM3IHFGtETchjGiqpLt

On the flip side, if levels dip below about 60–70 mg/dL, symptoms associated with low blood sugar, or hypoglycemia, start to set in. These include hunger and shakiness, and typically, if something is eaten immediately, the symptoms will disappear. However, without food, levels will dip even further, and they may go below about 50 mg/dL and continue to reduce drop further. If this happens, a medical emergency can develop due to continued loss of the patient's mental function, with eventual seizures and unconsciousness.

To learn more about hypoglycemia and its symptoms, visit:

http://www.nlm.nih.gov/medlineplus/ency/article/000386.htm

Regulating your blood sugar level is therefore extremely important for your body, because neither hyperglycemia nor hypoglycemia are good situations to be in. Keeping blood sugar levels within an ideal target range will help reduce your risk for developing the serious long-term health effects associated with diabetes. While there are recommended guidelines for blood sugar levels at different times of the day for people with diabetes, it is important to remember that they may not apply to everyone.

Table 3.1 Ideal blood sugar levels for people with diabetes

BEFORE A MEAL	70–130 MG/DL
1-2 hours after a meal	Less than 180 mg/dL

SOURCE: Based on the National Diabetes Information Clearinghouse's, "What should my blood glucose numbers be?"

http://diabetes.niddk.nih.gov/dm/pubs/complications_control/#numbers

If you have diabetes, your goals may be higher or lower than this, and your doctor will help you set your particular blood sugar target range.

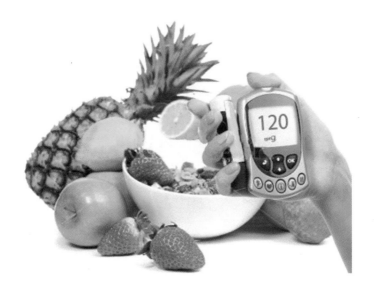

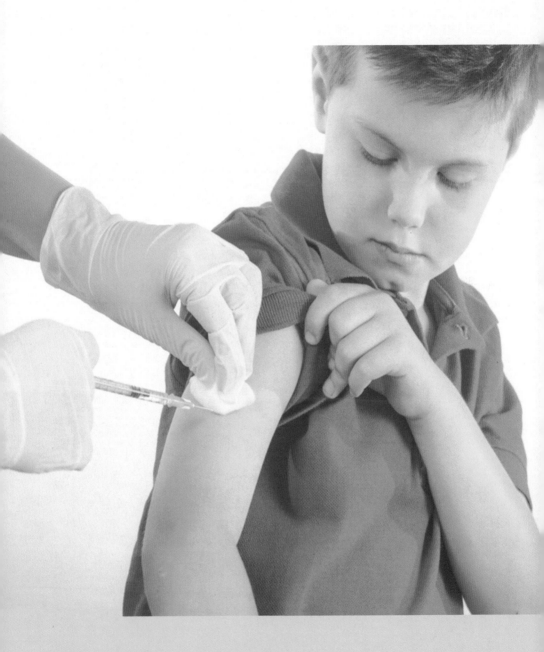

PART TWO

Causes, Effects, and Risk Factors for Diabetes

In Part Two, we will discuss more about how the pancreas relates to diabetes. We will answer questions about type 1 and type 2 diabetes, discussing what they are, what causes them, and who is at risk for each type. Finally, we will take a look at some cases of secondary diabetes. This may occur in some special circumstances, including during pregnancy, when taking certain drugs, and in association with other diseases such as hormonal disorders or pancreatic injury.

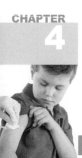

How Does the Pancreas Relate to Diabetes?—Type 1 Diabetes

10. What is type 1 diabetes?

Type 1 diabetes, also previously known as juvenile diabetes or insulin-dependent diabetes, is the less common form of the 2 types of diabetes, and occurs because the pancreas stops producing insulin due to permanent destruction of the beta cells.

DEFINITION

See how type 1 diabetes results when the pancreas stops making insulin:

ON THE WEB

http://www.youtube.com/watch?v=_OOWhuC_9Lw

Type 1 diabetes is a condition that arises because the body is no longer able to produce enough insulin, which leads to problems regulating blood sugar levels. In type 1 diabetes, cells can no longer take up sugar from the bloodstream in the normal way to use it for energy. And as a result, there is too much sugar in the bloodstream—a condition known as hyperglycemia. The symptoms of type 1 diabetes typically become evident when approximately 90% of the beta cells have been destroyed. So this means that the destruction of the beta cells can take place over a long period of time, often many years, but the symptoms will develop over a short period of time once about 80% of the tissue is affected.

11. What causes type 1 diabetes?

Type 1 diabetes is a very complex disease that has nothing to do with diet or lifestyle. It is considered to be a progressive, inflammatory, autoimmune disorder—a disease that occurs when the body's immune system attacks and destroys the body's own healthy tissues. In type 1 diabetes, the immune system slowly attacks beta cells in the pancreas that make insulin. The islet cells that make the other hormones are typically spared in this disease, although they may be redistributed within the islets. Although the exact reason for the autoimmune attack on the beta cells remains unknown, research has shown that numerous factors may contribute to its development. However, type 1 diabetes cannot be prevented or cured.

Genetics is also an important contributing factor. The risk of type 1 diabetes has been shown to be associated with certain types of the genes that belong to a family called the **human leukocyte antigen (HLA) complex**. This complex helps the immune system to be able to differentiate the body's own proteins from those made by foreign invaders like bacteria and viruses. People have a specific combination of different types of these HLA genes, known as a haplotype. And certain HLA haplotypes are major risk genes for type 1 diabetes, with particular combinations of genes known as *HLA-DQA1*, *HLA-DQB1*, and *HLA-DRB1* resulting in the highest risk. These genes provide instructions to allow the body to make proteins that play an important role in the immune system. HLA variations account for about 40% of the genetic risk for type 1 diabetes. But although people with these specific HLA haplotypes seem to have a higher risk of the pancreatic beta cells being attacked by the immune system, it is important to note that only about 5% of these people go on to develop the disease.

▼ **FIGURE 4.1**
Beta Cells in the Pancreas in Type 1 Diabetes.

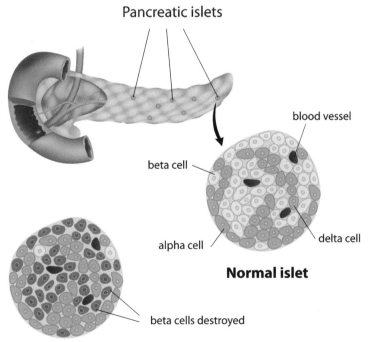

Pancreatic islets

blood vessel

beta cell

alpha cell

delta cell

Normal islet

beta cells destroyed

Type 1 diabetes

SOURCE: Shutterstock, Inc.

For more information about some of the factors that influence the development of type 1 diabetes, visit:

http://ghr.nlm.nih.gov/condition/type-1-diabetes

Exposure to some viruses has also been suggested to increase the odds of type 1 diabetes developing in people with genetic risk factors. Viruses such as coxsackievirus B, Epstein-Barr virus, adenovirus, rubella virus, cytomegalovirus, and mumps virus may directly infect the beta cells, or trigger autoimmune destruction of them.

Although diet itself does not cause the disease, some research has shown that it may contribute to type 1 diabetes risk. One study looked at children who were at increased risk of type 1 diabetes because they had first-degree relatives with the disease. And it was found that those who were given solid food for the first time either earlier or later than other children had a higher risk of type 1 diabetes. The risk was increased in children who were exposed earlier to fruit, and later to oats and rice. The risk was lower in children exposed to wheat or barley when they were still being breastfed. This study suggested that, in high-risk children, the best time to introduce solid foods is between 4 and 5 months of age, and that solid foods are best introduced while children are still being breastfed.

To learn more about some of the causes of type 1 diabetes, see: Document 4.1.CausesT1D.

http://physrev.physiology.org/content/91/1/79.full.pdf+html
Document 4.2.GeneticsT1D

http://www.intechopen.com/books/type-1-diabetes-pathogenesis-genetics-and-immunotherapy/relationship-of-type-1-diabetes-with-human-leukocyte-antigen-hla-class-ii-antigens-except-for-dr3-an

12. Who is at risk for type 1 diabetes?

Type 1 diabetes typically arises during childhood or adolescence, usually before the age of 25 years, and accounts for about 95% of cases of diabetes in patients in this age group. However, it can also arise later in adults. The disease is much less common than type 2 diabetes, and accounts for about 5 to 10% of cases of diabetes worldwide. However, as with type 2 diabetes, its incidence has tripled in the United States over the past 40 years. Type 1 diabetes costs the United States almost $15 billion every year in health care, with about 3 million Americans thought to have the disease. For reasons that are not completely clear, the risk of type 1 diabetes is higher in Caucasians than any other race, and the risk is much lower in Asians.

Males and females are equally at risk. And although type 1 diabetes is not an inherited disease, there is some genetic component involved. Family history is a risk factor in its development. The risk of developing type 1 diabetes increases 10 to 20 times if an immediate relative (such as a parent, son, daughter, brother, or sister) has the disease. If one child in the family has the disease, there is a 1 in 10 chance that their siblings will develop it by age 50 years. And children are more likely to inherit type 1 diabetes from a father with the disease, than a mother.

Other risk factors include:
- Being ill in early infancy
- Having an older mother
- Having a mother who had preeclampsia during pregnancy
- Having another autoimmune disorder such as multiple sclerosis, Hashimoto's thyroiditis, or Graves disease

Nevertheless, most people who develop type 1 diabetes have no family history of the disease, and genetic factors alone cannot explain its development. Additional things, such as environmental factors and other gene variations are also thought to affect the development of this complex disorder.

For more information about the incidence of type 1 diabetes, see: Document 4.3.IncidenceT1D

http://www.ncbi.nlm.nih.gov/pmc/articles/PMC2925303/pdf/nihms210033.pdf

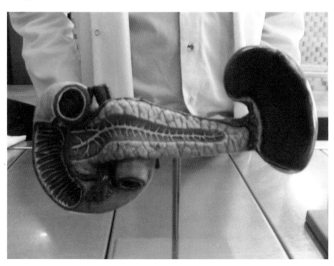

CHAPTER 5

How Does the Pancreas Relate to Diabetes?—Type 2 Diabetes

13. What is type 2 diabetes?

Type 2 diabetes, previously known as **adult-onset diabetes**, **maturity-onset diabetes**, and **noninsulin-dependent diabetes**, is the most common type of diabetes. It is a disease in which there is too much sugar in the bloodstream. And although the symptoms of type 2 diabetes can be successfully managed by a combination of weight loss, a healthy diet, and regular exercise, most patients have this disease for life.

In the United States alone, type 2 diabetes accounts for about 95% of all cases of diabetes. And it is estimated that 1 in 8 Americans has been diagnosed with the disease—about 29 million people. Type 2 diabetes is a serious condition that puts patients at risk for early death, and can even reduce lifespan by about 10 years. This is mostly due to some of the life-threatening complications that go along with it, such as the increased risk of heart disease and stroke, lower-limb amputations, and hospitalizations.

For a video explaining how type 2 diabetes affects your sugar levels, visit:

ON THE WEB

http://www.mayoclinic.org/condition/diabetes/multimedia/blood-sugar/vid-20084642

14. What causes type 2 diabetes?

Unlike in type 1 diabetes, people with type 2 diabetes do make insulin, the hormone that usually helps to take sugar from the bloodstream into the cells where it is needed for energy. The disease occurs either because the pancreas does not make enough insulin, or the body cannot use insulin properly (this is called **insulin resistance**). In both instances, sugar builds up in the blood when it is not taken into the body's cells, and so the cells do not function properly. The build-up of sugar in the bloodstream also leads to damage in many parts of the body, like the kidneys, heart, and eyes.

Despite being the more common type of diabetes, the exact causes of type 2 diabetes are still not fully understood. Contrary to what some people believe, type 2 diabetes is not caused by eating too many sweet foods and drinks. Many things are likely involved in contributing to the development of this disease, including genetics, family history, and lifestyle.

15. Who is at risk for type 2 diabetes?

Type 2 diabetes is most common in adults. While anyone can get this disease, some people have a higher risk, and it is most often associated with:

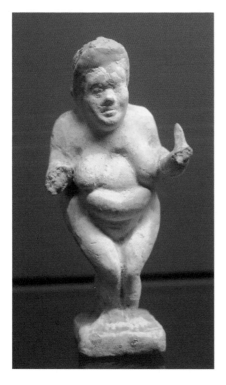

- Being overweight or obese
- Lack of exercise
- Prediabetes
- High blood pressure
- Low levels of high density lipid (HDL) cholesterol or high levels of triglycerides
- A family history of diabetes
- Increasing age (over 45 years)
- Certain races

There are 2 main categories of risk factors associated with type 2 diabetes—uncontrollable factors that you cannot change (like your age, health history, family history, and race), and controllable factors, namely your lifestyle choices, that you can change.

Although not everyone with type 2 diabetes is overweight, the two most common causes of this disease are obesity and lack of exercise, and about 80% of affected patients are overweight or obese. In particular, abdominal obesity, or increased fat around the belly area and around the internal organs, increases

For more information on what can increase your risk for type 2 diabetes, visit:

http://diabetes.niddk.nih.gov/dm/pubs/riskfortype2/#7

your risk of type 2 diabetes. One easy way to assess your level of abdominal obesity, and therefore determine your risk of type 2 diabetes in this area, is to measure your waist. This reflects how much abdominal fat you have. Abdominal fat has been shown to interfere with the body's ability to react to insulin, and consists of the fat under the skin around your belly (subcutaneous fat) and fat around your internal organs (visceral fat).

The two kinds of body fat

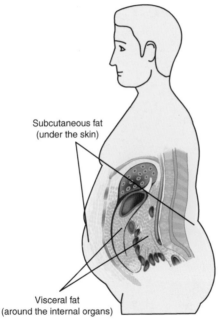

Subcutaneous fat
(under the skin)

Visceral fat
(around the internal organs)

SOURCE: Illustration adapted from www.zestzfulness.blogspot.com

◀ FIGURE 5.1
Distribution of Different Types of Fat Around the Abdomen.

Research has shown that waist size is strongly linked to type 2 diabetes, especially in women.

The risk of type 2 diabetes is increased if you are a:

- Woman with a waist measurement of 31.5 inches or more
- Asian man with a waist measurement of 35 inches or more
- White or black man with a waist measurement of 37 inches or more

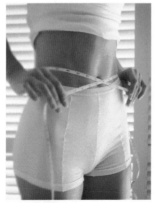

In people with prediabetes, modest weight loss (about 5%–7% of bodyweight) and regular exercise (about 2 and a half hours of brisk walking each week) have been shown to help guard against the development of type 2 diabetes by more than 50%.

Drinking large amounts of alcohol can also damage the pancreas and contribute to development of type 2 diabetes. Alcohol intake should be limited to a maximum of one drink daily for women and 2 drinks daily for men.

Smokers are also much more likely than non-smokers to develop type 2 diabetes, because smoking can also damage the pancreas. If you are a smoker, you should take immediate steps to stop, in order to lower your chances of developing type 2 diabetes and other serious health problems.

While type 2 diabetes often arises in white people over the age of 45, people of African, African-Caribbean, South Asian, and Middle Eastern descent have a higher chance of developing it when they are much younger.

The frequency of type 2 diabetes is now also rising in children, especially due to the increase in childhood obesity, with about 3,600 new cases diagnosed each year. Among children, type 2 diabetes is most common in American Indian youth. It is also becoming more and more common in African-American, Pacific Islander, and Mexican-American children.

The National Diabetes Prevention Program offers a lifestyle change program to help prevent or delay the development of type 2 diabetes. To learn more about this program, visit:

http://www.cdc.gov/diabetes/prevention/about.htm

And to see if there is a program offered in your area, visit:

http://www.cdc.gov/diabetes/prevention/recognition/registry.htm

To see if you are at risk for type 2 diabetes, take this quick online questionnaire:

http://www.diabetes.org/are-you-at-risk/diabetes-risk-test/

As the number of people with type 2 diabetes continues to rise, so will the financial burden to society due to the cost of managing the disease. In addition to direct costs to the health care sector, people with the disease are also burdened with heavy medical costs. One study estimated that a patient between 25 and 44 years of age diagnosed with type 2 diabetes is likely to spend more than $120,000 in health care costs over his or her lifetime. More than half of this cost accounts for treating the complications of the disease. These costs are increased the earlier in life the disease is diagnosed.

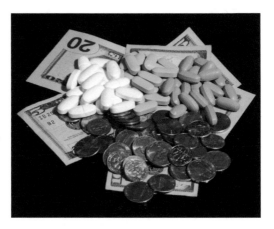

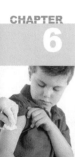

CHAPTER

6 *Some Other Forms of Diabetes*

16. Why do some women develop diabetes during pregnancy?

It is normal for most women to develop a small degree of insulin resistance and impaired glucose tolerance during late pregnancy (gestation). But a small number of women who have never had diabetes before can develop high blood sugar levels. This is known as **gestational diabetes** or **diabetes of pregnancy**.

For a video explaining what gestational diabetes is, visit:

http://www.thevisualmd.com /center.php?idg=8353

ON THE WEB

It is mostly a temporary condition, and occurs in less than 5% of pregnant women, and is typically diagnosed during the later stages of pregnancy.

Although the exact cause of gestational diabetes is not fully understood, it is thought to occur as a result of the changes that take place in a woman's body when she is pregnant. These changes are thought to lead to insulin resistance in some women.

Some women have a higher risk of gestational diabetes, and this can be associated with:

- Being overweight or obese
- Having prediabetes
- Having had gestational diabetes in a previous pregnancy
- Having previously given birth to a baby over 9 pounds
- Having a family history of type 2 diabetes
- Having polycystic ovary syndrome
- Being African-American, Asian-American, Hispanic, American Indian, or Pacific Islander-American

Gestational diabetes usually does not produce any symptoms, and it is typically diagnosed during routine screening during pregnancy, before it even gets the chance to cause any symptoms. However, if it happens to go undetected, occasionally, some women may feel more thirsty than normal, or feel the need to urinate more frequently.

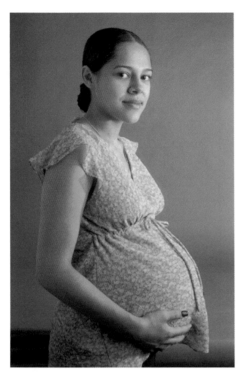

Screening tests for gestational diabetes are therefore important, and most women have a blood test to check for the condition between the 24th and 28th weeks of pregnancy. This time period is chosen because it is when the placenta is making a lot of hormones that may contribute to cause insulin resistance. The screening test involves the woman drinking a sugary drink, and then having her blood tested for sugar levels an hour later. If the results are abnormal, additional tests will be performed to confirm a diagnosis of gestational diabetes.

Women with gestational diabetes who receive the right medical care usually deliver healthy babies. But if gestational diabetes is untreated, the high blood sugar level in the mother will affect the developing baby. It can cause the baby to be bigger than normal, and this may lead to complications during birth—affected women have a higher chance of needing a Caesarian section delivery.

▼ FIGURE 6.1
How Glucose Affects the Developing Fetus.

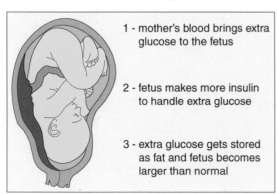

1 - mother's blood brings extra glucose to the fetus

2 - fetus makes more insulin to handle extra glucose

3 - extra glucose gets stored as fat and fetus becomes larger than normal

SOURCE: adapted from www.lifemartini.com

Other potential problems for the baby include:

- Low blood sugar after birth
- Jaundice
- Respiratory distress syndrome

For additional information on gestational diabetes, see:

ON THE DVD

Document 6.1.GDMBooklet

http://diabetes.niddk.nih.gov/dm/pubs
/gestational/gestationaldm.pdf

Document 6.2.GDMArticle

http://care.diabetesjournals.org/content/26/
suppl_1/s103.full.pdf+html

For more information on what you need to know about diet if you have diabetes, visit:

ON THE WEB

http://diabetes.niddk.nih.gov/dm/pubs
/eating_ez/index.aspx

- Death before or after birth
- Becoming overweight and developing type 2 diabetes later in life

But the good news is that the risk of problems associated with gestational diabetes is reduced when women receive the appropriate treatment, so it is important to follow your doctor's advice during this time. Healthy eating is the main approach to managing this condition, and this allows many women to control their sugar levels adequately. Your doctor can also advise you on an exercise plan, if necessary. However, in some cases, diet and exercise alone may not be enough to control your blood sugar levels, and insulin therapy may be needed.

For women with gestational diabetes, blood sugar levels usually return to normal soon after birth. However, affected women will be at risk for developing type 2 diabetes, so it is important to continue to work with your doctor to monitor and control your blood sugar.

17. What is drug-induced diabetes?

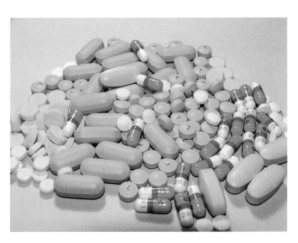

Drug-induced diabetes occurs when the use of certain non−diabetes-related medications leads to the development of diabetes in patients who have never had diabetes before. This is a form of secondary diabetes, which means diabetes that has arisen due to having another health condition. Drugs can induce diabetes in different ways. Some interfere with insulin production and release by the pancreas, while others interfere with the action of insulin.

Numerous medications have been linked with an increased risk of developing type 2 diabetes. These include:

- *Corticosteroids:* These are powerful drugs used to treat various conditions, including inflammation and autoimmune diseases. Usually the increased blood sugar levels return to normal after a short course of treatment is ended. But sometimes, especially if they are taken for a long time, type 2 diabetes may result and be permanent.
- *Beta blockers:* These drugs, such as atenolol, are used to help reduce heart rate and blood pressure, and are often used to treat patients with high blood pressure, angina, and heart disease.
- *Thiazide diuretics:* These "water tablets" are often taken by patients who need to remove excess water from the body or by some patients with high blood pressure.
- *Other drugs to control high blood pressure:* These include angiotensin receptor blockers (ARBs), angiotensin converting enzyme (ACE) inhibitors, and calcium channel blockers (CCBs).
- *Statins:* These drugs are commonly used to help lower high cholesterol levels.
- *Immunosuppressive drugs:* Drugs like cyclosporine and tacrolimus, for example, may be used in organ transplant patients, to help reduce the chances of their body rejecting the transplanted organ.
- *Antipsychotic drugs:* Drugs like clozapine and olanzapine may be used to treat schizophrenia and symptoms of psychosis that can occur in patients with dementia.

Drug-induced diabetes is not always permanent. Blood sugar levels may return to normal after the medication is stopped, but sometimes the diabetes can be permanent, especially in cases where significant weight gain has occurred during the course of treatment.

ON THE DVD

To read more about corticosteroid-induced diabetes, see Document 6.3.SteroidDiab:

http://www.ccjm.org/content/78/11/748.full.pdf+html

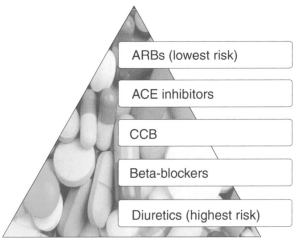

ARBs (lowest risk)

ACE inhibitors

CCB

Beta-blockers

Diuretics (highest risk)

SOURCE: Illustration adapted from www.medindia.net

If you have developed drug-induced diabetes, your doctor will be able to advise you on how to manage this condition. If you can stop taking the medication that caused the problem, or even take a smaller dose, your blood sugar levels may be easier to control. However, this may not be possible. If you do need to continue taking the medication that brought on the diabetes, you may find it harder to manage your diabetes. Your doctor will be able to advise you on following a healthy diet and getting regular exercise to help the situation. And in some cases, he or she may recommend also taking diabetes medication, including insulin.

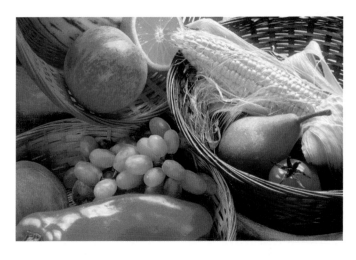

Diabetes itself results from a hormonal imbalance, because it results from an imbalance of insulin, which eventually leads to an inability to control blood sugar levels. The body produces a lot of hormones, and they all work together and influence each other. So when there is an imbalance in any of these other hormones, it can affect the levels or effectiveness of insulin in the body.

In women, for example, this can be especially obvious around the time of menopause. During perimenopause, a woman's progesterone levels become lowered. This leads to problems dealing with insulin, and eventually results in insulin resistance.

In patients with Cushing's syndrome, raised levels of cortisol, the stress hormone made by the adrenal glands, can also result in insulin resistance. Diabetes can then also cause the adrenal glands to make even more cortisol, which can keep the cycle going.

Hyperthyroidism, a hormonal condition where the thyroid gland makes too much thyroid hormone, can also lead to increased blood sugar levels due to insulin resistance or sugar intolerance.

Cortisol mostly comes from the adrenal gland, but some also comes from the brain, liver and fat

Adrenal   Brain   Liver   Fat

↑Cortisol

Muscle:
↓glucose uptake

Fat:
↑fat deposition

Liver:
↑glucose generation

Brain:
↑food intake

Diabetes

Pancreas:
↑Insulin release

Obesity

SOURCE: Illustration adapted from
www.whitegroup.ls.manchester.ac.uk

◀ FIGURE 6.3
The Effect of Cortisol on Different Tissues of the Body.

ON THE DVD

To learn more about the link between thyroid disease and diabetes, see Document 6.4.ThyT1D

http://www.ncbi.nlm.nih.gov/pmc/articles/PMC3139205/pdf/JTR2011-439463.pdf

To read more about different types of secondary diabetes, see Document 6.5.SecT1D

http://diabetes.niddk.nih.gov/dm/pubs/america/pdf/chapter5.pdf

Acromegaly is another hormonal condition that can lead to diabetes. It is a condition in which the body's pituitary gland produces too much growth hormone. This in turn can lead to insulin resistance or sugar intolerance.

19. How does injury to the pancreas cause diabetes?

Although rare, it is possible for type 1 diabetes to result from physical injury to the pancreas, such as trauma to the abdominal region. The pancreas is vulnerable to physical injury due to crushing against the spinal column. In these rare cases, the trauma leads to inflammation of the pancreas, known as **pancreatitis**. If this is severe and a large area is involved, the pancreas can be destroyed due to inflammation and scarring, and this can lead to diabetes.

The development of diabetes as a severe complication of trauma to the abdomen is reported to occur in less than 1% of cases. In children, bicycle accidents are a common cause of pancreatic injury, due to the handlebars crushing the abdomen. In adults, motor vehicle accidents are the most common cause, due to a misplaced seatbelt or the steering wheel crushing the abdominal region.

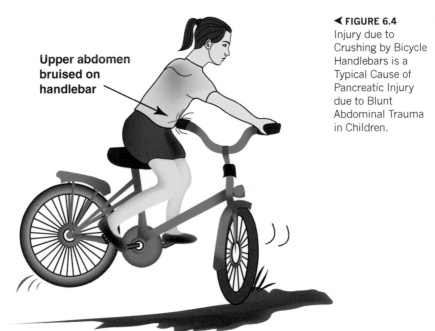

Upper abdomen bruised on handlebar

◄ FIGURE 6.4
Injury due to Crushing by Bicycle Handlebars is a Typical Cause of Pancreatic Injury due to Blunt Abdominal Trauma in Children.

SOURCE: Illustration adapted from www.rcsed.ac.uk

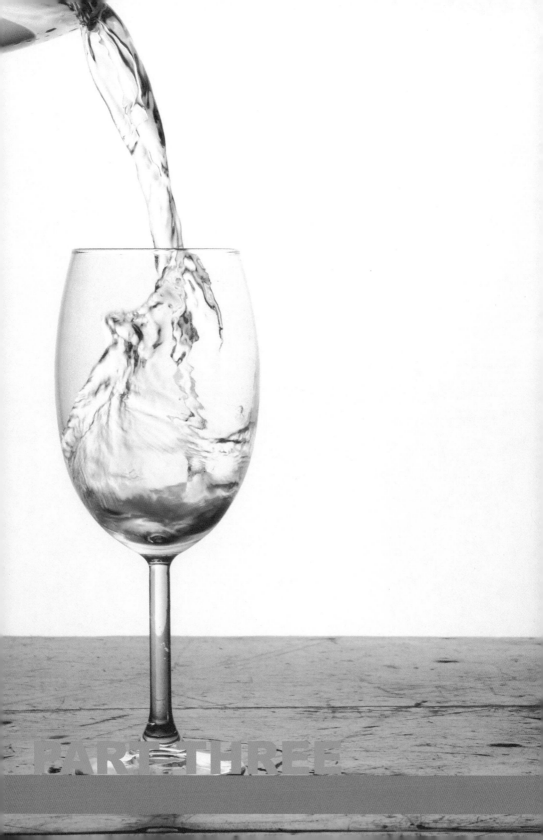

PART THREE

Symptoms and Diagnosis of Diabetes

In Part Three, we will focus on the symptoms of diabetes. We will answer questions about the symptoms of type 1 diabetes and type 2 diabetes, discussing their similarities and differences. We will also take a look at how other medical conditions with similar symptoms can sometimes be mistaken for diabetes. Finally we will discuss how diabetes is diagnosed, in particular covering what diagnostic tests are used, who should be screened, and how test results can help determine if you have prediabetes.

CHAPTER 7

Symptoms of Diabetes, Including Increased Hunger and Increased Thirst

CHAPTER 8

Diagnosis of Diabetes

Symptoms of Diabetes, Including Increased Hunger and Increased Thirst

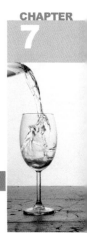

20. What are the symptoms of type 1 diabetes?

Although type 1 diabetes can occur at any age, it is most commonly diagnosed in children.

There are numerous symptoms of type 1 diabetes. Some of the more common ones, which may develop quickly, include:

- **Excessive thirst:** This occurs because you become dehydrated due to water loss.
- **More frequent urination:** The kidneys must work extra hard to get rid of the excess sugar that has built up in the bloodstream. The excess sugar must be flushed out along with water, so this leads to more frequent urination. This is also what leads to the dehydration and excessive thirst.
- **Unexpected weight loss:** This occurs because your body can no longer make use of the sugar in the blood. So when it is lost in the urine, this means you are losing all the calories from sugar in your food. Patients often notice weight loss even though they are eating their normal amount of food. The dehydration can also contribute to weight loss. Unexpected weight loss is one of the common symptoms in women especially.
- **Increased hunger:** You may be more hungry than usual, even though your activity level has not changed. This is because your body cannot make use of the sugar in your food, and you are losing its valuable calories as it is eliminated in the urine.
- **Unusual tiredness:** Because you are losing so much sugar in your urine, you are losing out on the calories that provide you with energy. As a result you may feel more tired than usual, even though your activity level has not changed.

- **Blurred vision:** When excess sugar builds up in the blood, it can also build up in the lens of the eye. This pulls extra water into the lens too, and causes the lens to change shape. This leads to blurry vision.

To learn more about the warning signs of type 1 diabetes, see Document 7.1.SignsT1D

ON THE DVD

http://cdn.jdrf.org/wp-content/uploads/2012/12/WarningSigns.pdf

Any number of these symptoms can be present in association with type 1 diabetes, and as time goes on, they become more pronounced, or more symptoms may also appear.

Listen to how type 1 diagnosis was diagnosed in one child:

ON THE WEB

http://www.youtube.com/watch?v=_OOWhuC_9Lw

Some other less frequent symptoms include:

- Dry skin and mouth
- Nausea and vomiting
- Slow-healing sores
- Repeated vaginal infections in women
- Yeast infections in women and men
- Itchy skin
- Numbness and tingling in the feet

21. What are the symptoms of type 2 diabetes?

Type 2 diabetes is sometimes called a "silent disease." This is because many people have type 2 diabetes and don't know about it. They may have symptoms for years without a diagnosis, until some complication develops, like heart disease. Often there are no symptoms associated with type 2 diabetes.

More often this diagnosis is made through routine screening tests performed by a physician. But when symptoms do occur, the more common ones may be similar to those in type 1 diabetes, although they tend to develop more slowly in type 2 diabetes:

To learn more about the symptoms of type 2 diabetes, visit:

ON THE WEB

http://www.dlife.com/diabetes/type-2/symptoms

- **Excessive thirst**
- **More frequent urination**
- **Unexpected weight loss—** but more commonly **weight gain**
- **Unusual tiredness**

Just like in type 1 diabetes, the following symptoms may occur, although they may be less common than those previously listed for type 2 diabetes:

- Dry skin and mouth
- Nausea and vomiting
- Slow-healing sores
- Repeated vaginal infections in women
- Yeast infections in women and men
- Itchy skin
- Numbness and tingling in the feet

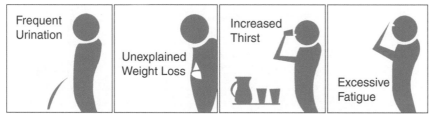

CLASSIC DIABETES SIGNS YOU MUST NOT MISS!

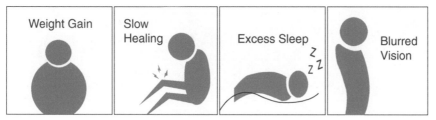

▲ **FIGURE 7.1**
Some Classic Signs of Diabetes.
SOURCE: Illustration adapted from www.healthkart.com

One particular warning sign that usually signifies type 2 diabetes is a condition known as **acanthosis nigricans**. This is a skin condition in which patches of dark, thickened skin occur around joints and in areas of the body with folds and creases, like the neck, knees, armpits, and elbows. It can occur in other areas too, however. The skin typically stays soft, and is often described as being velvety. It occurs because something (high levels of insulin in the case of type 2 diabetes) triggers the cells on the surface of the skin to increase in number. These new cells have more of the brown skin pigment called melanin. So this causes affected areas of the skin to appear darker.

To learn more about acanthosis nigricans, visit:

ON THE WEB

http://www.nlm.nih.gov/medlineplus/ency/article/000852.htm

Anyone can develop acanthosis nigricans, but it is more common in people of Hispanic, Caribbean, and African descent. Up to 75% of children with type 2 diabetes are reported to develop this condition.

Learn about the warning signs of type 2 diabetes:

http://www.youtube.com/watch?v=AVJwcwbL054

ON THE WEB

Although the discoloration and thickening may never completely go away, getting the symptoms of diabetes under control, and losing weight if necessary, can reduce the appearance of the condition.

22. Can other conditions be mistaken for diabetes?

Although the more common symptoms will usually lead your physician to immediately want to check for diabetes, many of these symptoms do not just occur in diabetes, and can occur in other conditions too. Some conditions may share some of the symptoms most commonly seen with diabetes.

Table 7.1 Some conditions with symptoms like diabetes

THIRST OR URINATION	WEIGHT LOSS	TIREDNESS
Chronic kidney failure	Chronic kidney failure	Heart disease
Chronic liver failure (cirrhosis)	Chronic liver failure (cirrhosis)	Lung diseases like COPD
Hormonal conditions like Cushing's syndrome	Hormonal conditions like hyperthyroidism	Hormonal conditions like hypothyroidism
Chemical substances like diuretic pills and caffeine	Intestinal conditions like Crohn's disease	Intestinal conditions like Crohn's disease
Kidney or bladder infection	Lifestyle choices like heavy smoking or drug abuse	Lyme disease
Prostate disease	Cancer	Cancer
Anxiety and depression	Anxiety and depression	Anxiety and depression

Table 7.1 Continued

THIRST OR URINATION	WEIGHT LOSS	TIREDNESS
Pregnancy		Insomnia and sleep apnea
Dehydration		Multiple sclerosis
		Chronic fatigue syndrome
		Anemia
		Medications like antihistamines and cold remedies
		Obesity

Acanthosis nigricans: Although acanthosis nigricans is more likely to indicate type 2 diabetes, it can also occur in other conditions that may affect the body's insulin levels, such as:

- Hypothyroidism
- Addison's disease
- Diseases of the pituitary gland
- Cancer of the liver or stomach

It can also occur in association with medications, such as:

- Birth control pills
- Growth hormone therapy
- Thyroid medications

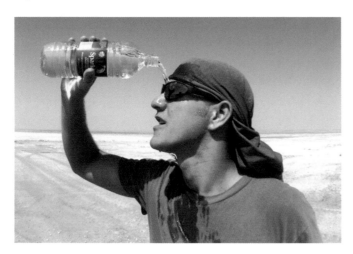

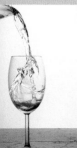

CHAPTER 8 *Diagnosis of Diabetes*

23. Who should be screened for diabetes?

Screening tests for diabetes are important because many people have type 2 diabetes but don't realize it. Since the symptoms of type 1 diabetes develop quickly and are usually noticeable, screening recommendations typically focus on type 2 diabetes.

According to the American Diabetes Association, everyone 45 years and older should be tested for diabetes. If the results are normal, they should then be tested every 3 years to recheck.

However, people with certain diabetes risk factors need to be tested earlier in life and more frequently. These risk factors include:

- Being overweight (if BMI is higher than 25)
- A family history of diabetes
- People of high-risk ethnicities (African-American, Asian-American, Native American, Hispanic-American, or Pacific Islander)
- High blood pressure
- High HDL cholesterol or triglyceride levels
- A history of gestational diabetes or giving birth to a baby over 9 pounds
- Impaired glucose tolerance or impaired fasting tolerance when previously tested

To learn more about the risk factors for diabetes, visit:

ON THE WEB

http://ndep.nih.gov/am-i-at-risk/DiabetesRiskFactors.aspx

24. What tests will my doctor use to diagnose whether I have diabetes?

There are various tests that can help your doctor make a diagnosis of diabetes. Initially your doctor will take a blood sample from you, and order a fasting blood glucose test or a casual blood glucose test.

Fasting plasma glucose: Your doctor will schedule a time for this test, and you will not be able to eat or drink anything (except water) for 8 hours before it. This is usually done in the morning.

Casual glucose: Your doctor will take a blood sample from you at any time when you have severe symptoms of diabetes, regardless of whether or not you have eaten recently. In a person without diabetes, blood sugar levels should not vary much throughout the day. And even after a meal, sugar levels do not change very much in a person without diabetes. But in people with diabetes, blood sugar levels are always high, and rise even higher just after eating. In people with prediabetes, blood sugar may rise higher than normal after eating, and often take longer to come back down than in people who do not have prediabetes or diabetes.

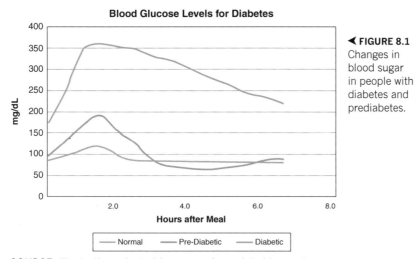

◀ FIGURE 8.1
Changes in blood sugar in people with diabetes and prediabetes.

SOURCE: Illustration adapted from www.foyupdate.blogspot.com

There are also other tests that can be performed to check for diabetes:

Oral glucose tolerance test (OGTT): For people who have normal blood glucose levels, but risk factors for diabetes, or symptoms of diabetes, an oral glucose tolerance test may be used to make sure type 2 diabetes is not present. It measures how well the body can handle sugar.

Your doctor will schedule a time for this test, and you will not be able to eat or drink anything (except water) for at least 10 hours before it. This is usually done in the morning. For this test, a fasting blood sample will first be taken. Next, the patient will be given a sugary drink. More blood samples will then be taken at 30 to 60 minute intervals, usually for 2 hours. The before-and-after levels of sugar in the samples (see Table 8.2) will be compared to check if the body was able to process it properly.

For more information on the OGTT, visit:

http://www.nlm.nih.gov/medlineplus/ency/article/003466.htm

ON THE WEB

This test is also used in pregnant women after 24 weeks of pregnancy to check for gestational diabetes, and blood samples are taken at 1-, 2-, and 3-hours after a sugary drink. If 2 or more of the test results are higher than normal, this indicates a diagnosis of gestational diabetes.

Table 8.1 OGTT results in women with gestational diabetes

GLUCOSE TEST	RESULT
Fasting plasma glucose	95mg/dL or higher
1-hour after a sugary drink	180mg/dL or higher
2-hours after a sugary drink	155mg/dL or higher
3-hours after a sugary drink	140mg/dL or higher

Home monitoring tests: If you have been diagnosed with diabetes, you will continue to monitor your blood sugar level at home to monitor how well your treatment is working. You will do this by testing your blood sugar and/or your hemoglobin A1c (**HbA1c**) levels, as discussed more in Chapter 9.

HbA1c: A sample of blood is taken at any time. The level of glycosylated hemoglobin in the blood is measured. This provides a picture of average blood sugar levels—and therefore blood sugar control—over the past 2–3 months.

According to the American Diabetes Association, diabetes is indicated by any one of the following results:

Table 8.2 Blood test results in people with diabetes

TEST	RESULT
Fasting plasma glucose	126mg/dL or higher
Casual plasma glucose	200mg/dL or higher
OGTT 2-hour blood sample	200mg/dL or higher
HbA1c	6.5% or more

There are various tests that can help your doctor make a diagnosis of prediabetes. Blood sugar screening can be performed in the same way as previously discussed for diabetes, using the fasting plasma glucose test, casual blood glucose test, OGTT, and HbA1c test.

To learn more about prediabetes testing visit:

http://www.thevisualmd.com/read_videoguide/?idu=1083609629&q=blood

Prediabetes is discussed more in Chapter 1. It is defined by any one of the following results:

Table 8.3 Blood test results in people with prediabetes

TEST	RESULT
Fasting plasma glucose	100–125mg/dL on 2 different occasions
Casual plasma glucose	140–199mg/dL
OGTT 2-hour blood sample	140–199mg/dL on 2 different occasions
HbA1c	5.7–6.4%

Prediabetes is diagnosed when blood sugar levels are in a "gray zone"—levels are higher than normal, but not high enough to be called diabetes.

For a screening test to check whether you could have prediabetes, see Document 8.1.ScreenPD

http://www.michigan.gov/documents/mdch/cdc-prediabetes-screening-test_400371_7.pdf

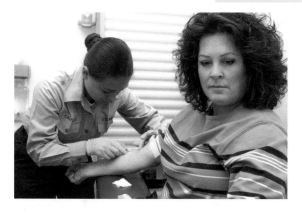

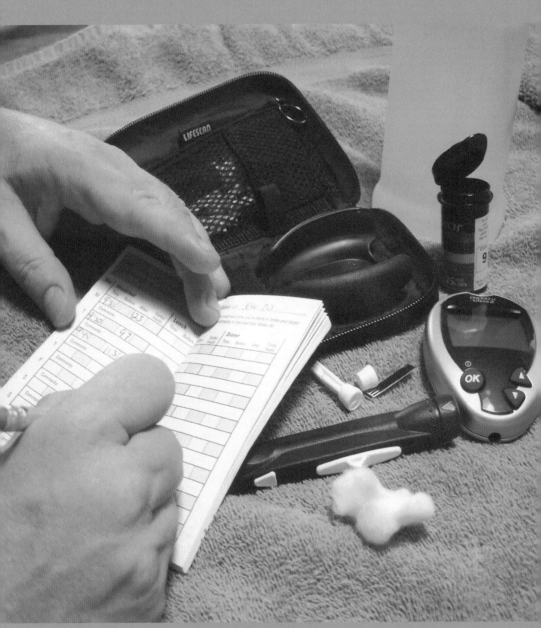

PART FOUR

Management of Diabetes

In Part Four, we will discuss blood sugar monitoring, in particular the use of a blood sugar meter and HbA1c testing. We will answer questions about some of the drugs commonly used to help control blood sugar, and then expand our discussion to insulin therapy, including the different types of insulin, and ways to administer it. We will also discuss some other drugs that may be required if you have diabetes, such as drugs to control cholesterol or high blood pressure. Finally, we will look at managing diabetes in some special cases, including children, pregnant women, and the elderly.

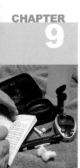

Monitoring Blood Sugar, Including the Use of a Blood Sugar Meter and HbA1c Testing

26. Why do I need to check my blood sugar levels?

If you have been diagnosed with diabetes, checking your blood sugar level is an important part of your treatment. The goal of treatment is to keep your blood sugar as close to normal as possible, so it is not too low and not too high. So, checking your blood sugar will help you manage your diabetes better, and this will help reduce your risk of diabetes complications. It will help you make the best choices throughout the day about your meals, your activity level, and how much medication you need. It will also help you know if your blood sugar is getting too low (hypoglycemia) or too high (hyperglycemia).

For more information on checking your blood sugar levels, visit:

http://www.cdc.gov/diabetes/pubs/tcyd/ktrack.htm#testing

ON THE WEB

27. Can I check my blood sugar levels at home?

Yes, you should be checking your blood sugar levels at home every day, especially if you are on multiple daily insulin injections or if you use an **insulin pump**. Ask your doctor how often you should check your blood sugar levels, because different diabetes healthcare specialists have different opinions on how frequently this should be done. Also, different people with diabetes have different needs. Your doctor or diabetes specialist can advise you based on your special circumstances. However, as a guide, many people with diabetes may check their blood sugar levels 4 to 6 times per day:

- When they first wake up
- Before meals
- 1–2 hours after a meal
- Immediately before exercise
- Immediately after exercise

You may only need to check your blood sugar once or twice a day if your levels tend to stay in a healthy range, or if you do not need to take insulin.

However, you may need to check your blood sugar more frequently than 4 to 6 times each day in certain circumstances:

- When you start getting used to your diabetes treatment plan
- When you change diabetes medication
- When your eating or activity plans change
- If you are sick or stressed
- If your diabetes is not under control
- If you exercise heavily

For a copy of a blood sugar log sheet, see Document 9.1.BSLog

http://www.dhs.wisconsin.gov/publications/P0/P00246.pdf

28. What is a blood sugar meter?

A blood sugar meter is a small computerized machine (also known as a glucometer) you can carry with you that measures how much sugar is in your blood.

▼ FIGURE 9.1
A blood sugar meter.

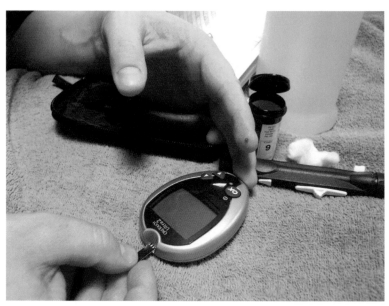

SOURCE: MorgueFile.

Using a blood sugar meter to test sugar levels will give an immediate reading of your blood sugar, and this helps you better manage your diabetes. It allows you to monitor for changes in your blood sugar that can be caused by things such as food, exercise, illness, and other medicines. Experts advise aiming to keep your blood sugar levels between 70 and 130 mg/dL before meals, and less than 180 mg/dL 1 to 2 hours after meals.

Most blood sugar meters come with test strips, small needles (lancets), and a log book for recording your sugar levels. To check your blood sugar level, you will first need to get a sample of your blood. You will clean the area where you will take the blood sample (usually the finger, but other locations are now being used, such as the palm of the hand or the forearm). Next you will use the lancet to pierce the skin, to draw a little blood. Then you apply the drop of blood to a test strip that is placed into the meter. The test strip contains a chemical to help determine how much sugar is in the blood. The meter will then measure how much sugar is present and display the level as a number on the screen after a few seconds.

See how to use a blood sugar meter as part of your diabetes care plan:

http://www.youtube.com/watch?v=rMMpeLLgdgY

ON THE WEB

There are many different blood sugar meters available, and your doctor or diabetes specialist will help you decide which one is best for you. But some features you should look for when you are choosing a blood sugar meter include:

- Its size
- What size blood sample it needs
- How quickly it gives you a reading
- How easy it is to read the numbers on the display screen
- What locations you can take your blood sample from
- Cost and insurance coverage
- How easy it is to use

29. Why is hemoglobin HbA1c testing also helpful from time to time?

Hemoglobin (Hb) is the pigment in red blood cells that transports oxygen. HbA1c is a specific type of this substance. Sugar in the blood attaches to HbA1c, producing glycosylated Hb. So the amount of HbA1c in the blood depends on how much sugar is in the blood. Once the sugar has attached to HbA1c, it stays there for about 3 months, until the red blood cell dies. Therefore, HbA1c gives you an idea of overall blood sugar control during the past 3 months or so.

Checking your blood sugar with a meter multiple times every day is useful to tell you how your blood sugar control is in the short term. This helps you regulate your sugar levels according to your with meals, exercise, and medications. But since you can't measure your sugar levels every minute of the day, this doesn't tell you much about what is happening during the times in between. This is where measuring HbA1c levels is helpful, because it tells you how your sugar control has been on average over a longer time period.

How often you need to have your HbA1c tested depends on your condition (see Table 9.1).

Table 9.1 How often to have your HbA1c levels tested

CONDITION	WHEN TO HAVE YOUR HbA1c TESTED
Type 1 diabetes	3 to 4 times a year
Type 2 diabetes: • But you don't use insulin • Blood sugar is usually in a healthy range	2 times a year
Type 2 diabetes: • And you use insulin • Blood sugar difficult to keep in a healthy range	4 times a year

30. What should my HbA1c level be?

The higher your HbA1c level, the higher your sugar level is. This means your blood sugar has not been controlled well, and you are at risk for diabetes complications.

There are specific levels of HbA1c that will help your doctor make a diagnosis of prediabetes or diabetes (See Table 9.2).

Table 9.2 Interpretation of HbA1c levels

HbA1c LEVEL	INTERPRETATION
Less than 5.7%	Normal
6.5% or more	Prediabetes
5.7 to 6.4%	Diabetes

Although a normal HbA1c level is one below 5.7%, this isn't necessarily the number you will have to aim for as you manage your diabetes. Target levels of HbA1c will vary in different patients. Some people will not require such tight control as others, depending on things such as their life expectancy and level of diabetes complications. While a level of 7% or less is often a common treatment target for many patients with diabetes, this may not be the best target for others. For someone at the end of their life expectancy, for example, a level of 7 to 8%, or even higher, may be appropriate, especially if they are having trouble controlling their blood sugar levels. Therefore your doctor or diabetes specialist will discuss your diabetes management plan with you, to help you keep your HbA1c levels in as healthy a range as possible for your situation.

▼ FIGURE 9.2
Guide to HbA1c levels.

Know Your HbA1c!
The blood test with a memory

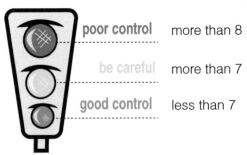

poor control — more than 8

be careful — more than 7

good control — less than 7

SOURCE: Illustration adapted from www.afmc.org

31. I've heard the term "eAG." What does this mean?

Your HbA1c level may be reported as an eAG level. This means "estimated average glucose" and refers to your average sugar level. Simply put, rather than giving you a percent value for your HbA1c level, your result has been converted a number in the same units as you usually see on your blood sugar meter. By providing the result as an eAG value, you will therefore be given a sugar level that will mean more to you.

32. What is the fructosamine test?

The fructosamine test is another blood test that can be used as a monitoring tool to help give you an idea of your blood sugar control. While HbA1c gives you an idea of blood sugar control over about a 3 month period, fructosamine gives you a picture of control over a short to intermediate time period—about 1 to 3 weeks. So if your fructosamine level is higher than normal, this means your blood sugar has not been controlled well for the past 1 to 3 weeks. The higher the fructosamine level, the poorer the blood sugar control.

▼ FIGURE 9.3
HbA1c levels and their corresponding eAG levels.

HbA1C%	eAGmg/dl
5	97
5.5	111
6	126
6.5	140
7	154
7.5	169
8	183
8.5	197
9	212
9.5	226
10	240
10.5	255
11	269
11.5	283
12	298

SOURCE: Illustration adapted from www.community.diabetes.org

This test is used to monitor blood sugar control—it cannot be used to screen for diabetes. It is often used in situations when changes in your blood sugar might occur quickly, so your doctor needs to monitor them. Some examples of these situations include times when you have had changes in your diabetes medication, or if you have gestational diabetes.

33. What are ketones, and why do I need to check for them?

Ketones are chemicals made by the body when there is not enough sugar to use as fuel. They are made in the liver when the body begins to burn fats for fuel. In people without diabetes, ketones are produced overnight, or in response to dieting or starvation. But in a person with diabetes, there is not enough insulin to allow the body to get sugar from the blood to use as energy. In this situation, the body starts to burn its own fat. If too much fat is burned, ketones may build up in the blood.

If you have diabetes, ketones can build up in different situations, like if you have not taken enough insulin, or if you missed a dose of insulin. It can also occur if you have eaten more food than you planned to eat. If ketones are allowed to build up and their levels continue to increase, this can result in a serious and life-threatening complication of diabetes known as diabetic keto-acidosis (DKA), which is described more in Chapter 14. Even if your diabetes is under control, this is an important test to know about. You should speak to your diabetes specialist about when to check for ketones, but you may be advised to test for them especially if:

- You feel sick
- You vomit
- You have abdominal pain
- Your blood sugar level is more than 300 mg/dL

For more information on when to check for ketones, and how the test is performed, visit:

ON THE WEB

http://www.nlm.nih.gov/medlineplus/ency/article/000320.htm

http://www.nlm.nih.gov/medlineplus/ency/article/003585.htm

Ketones can be tested in a urine sample or a blood sample. To test for ketones in urine, you use urine strips designed to measure ketones. The strip is first placed into a small sample of urine, and then you compare the color of the strip to the color chart on the bottle that contains the strips. Different color intensities indicate different ketone levels. Some of the newer blood sugar meters also now allow you to test for ketones.

34. How will I know if my blood sugar level is high?

In people with diabetes, blood sugar levels can be high (hypergly-cemia) for various reasons. They can be high if a dose of insulin has been skipped, or if you have eaten more food than planned. Other causes include problems with an insulin pump, or insulin that has been improperly stored, or may be out of date.

If your blood sugar levels are constantly higher than 200 mg/dL, you may start to have symptoms of high blood sugar.

Some of the warning signs of high blood sugar include:

- Feeling thirsty
- Urinating more than usual

- Feeling hungry
- Feeling tired
- Blurry vision
- Dry skin

However, some people with diabetes do not have any symptoms even when their blood sugar is this high. But if you do notice any of these symptoms, you should check your blood sugar level immediately so you can adjust your insulin dose.

35. What should I do if my blood sugar level is high?

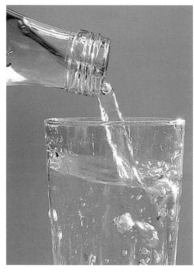

If you notice symptoms of high blood sugar, you should check your blood sugar levels. If the reading is high, you can adjust your insulin dose or meal plan accordingly, or check that your insulin pump is working, if you use one.

A single high blood sugar reading on its own usually isn't cause for alarm—it happens to everyone with diabetes at some point. But if you have numerous high blood sugar readings, or if you take insulin and your blood sugar level remains more than 200 mg/dL, you should seek medical help.

36. How will I know if my blood sugar level is low?

In people with diabetes, blood sugar levels can be low (hypoglycemia) for various reasons that may relate to your meal plan or diabetes medications, as discussed in Chapter 14. If your blood sugar levels are too low, typically less than 70 mg/dL, this becomes a problem. As your blood sugar level starts to gradually fall, you may start to have symptoms of low blood sugar.

Some of the early warning signs of low blood sugar include:

- Hunger
- Shakiness
- Sweatiness
- Irritability
- Headaches

If these early signs are ignored, the problem gradually worsens and can become a medical emergency. If blood sugar levels drop to about 40 mg/dL, this can lead to loss of consciousness and seizures in people with type 1 diabetes. If this is not treated immediately, it can lead to death.

37. What should I do if my blood sugar level is low?

If you notice symptoms of low blood sugar, you should check your blood sugar levels. If the reading is low, you need to eat or drink some sugar. This can be in the form of something like:

- Half a cup of fruit juice or soda (not diet versions)
- 4 to 6 pieces of hard candy
- 1 tablespoon of sugar, jam, or honey
- 3 glucose tablets

After 15 minutes, you should check your blood sugar level again. If it is still low, repeat the sugar treatment, and check again after another 15 minutes. When your blood sugar level has returned to normal, eat a small snack if your next meal is more than about 2 hours away.

In severe cases, if you lose consciousness or develop convulsions or seizures, for instance, emergency treatment is required.

Always check your blood sugar level before driving, especially if a long distance is involved. If the level is less than 100 mg/dL, eat a snack and recheck before getting behind the wheel. And don't forget to check regulations in your state, and anywhere else you are traveling, to make sure you are following the requirements for safe driving.

PRACTICAL TIP

For more detailed information on low blood sugar, see Document 9.2.LowBS

ON THE DVD

http://diabetes.niddk.nih.gov/dm/pubs/hypoglycemia/hypoglycemia_508.pdf

You should also discuss the problem with your diabetes specialist, so that your medications and meal plans can be adjusted, if necessary. And if you have an insulin pump, you should check to make sure it is in good working order. You should also always carry a sugar supply with you, wherever you go, so you are prepared for low blood sugar levels. And make sure friends and family know the warning signs of low blood sugar, and what they need to do if you should develop serious symptoms and cannot treat yourself.

Sugar control is the most important part of diabetes treatment. Ideally you want your blood sugar level to be as close to the normal range as possible, to reduce the risk of diabetic complications such as eye disease, kidney disease, and nerve disease.

For tight control, experts advise aiming to keep your blood sugar levels between 70 and 130 mg/dL before meals, and less than 180 mg/dL 1 to 2 hours after meals, with a target HbA1c level of less than 7%.

To do this, you need to pay strict attention to your eating and exercise, and to be aggressive with your insulin treatment. Because eating raises your blood sugar, and exercise lowers it, you have to play close attention to how these affect your blood sugar lev-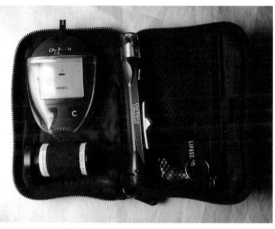els so you can plan your insulin treatment accordingly. Intensive insulin therapy is also needed, and this requires close monitoring of your blood sugar levels. The idea of the insulin routine is to mimic what happens in a person without diabetes. This means multiple injections of fast-acting insulin at mealtimes, and intermediate- or long-acting insulin at bedtime (these are discussed more in Chapter 11). You can also use an insulin pump to get the same result. You will need to check your blood sugar level multiple times each day, including before every injection, and about 2 or 3 hours after a meal to check for changes in blood sugar levels.

But controlling your blood sugar levels this tightly is hard work. Not everyone with diabetes wants to work this hard, and it may not even be necessary to get good results from your diabetes management. Additionally, there are problems associated with such a strict plan. People who practice tight control of their blood sugar are also more at risk for developing low blood sugar, and this can be just as problematic as high blood sugar. Many patients also experience weight gain from this intensive insulin regimen, and this can affect blood pressure and cholesterol levels, increasing risk factors for heart disease. Tight control using intensive insulin therapy can also be more expensive.

You should speak with your diabetes specialist to decide on a diabetes control plan that suits your individual situation. They can help you plan your exercise, keep a healthy weight, eat sensibly, and maintain reasonable blood sugar control.

Pills to Help Control Blood Sugar Levels, Including Metformin, Sulfonylurea Drugs, and Others

39. When are pills used to help control blood sugar?

In people with type 1 diabetes, the beta cells in the pancreas no longer make insulin. These patients must therefore receive insulin therapy for life. Insulin is not available in pill form because if taken by mouth, this would be broken down in the digestive system by chemicals that break down proteins. So insulin can only be given by injection.

But in people with type 2 diabetes, insulin is still produced by the pancreas. The problem in this condition is that either the insulin is not very effective at controlling blood sugar, or too little insulin is produced. In patients with type 2 diabetes, the first treatment involves lifestyle changes—diet, weight control, and exercise. If blood sugar remains high despite these changes, then pills are used to reduce sugar levels. These pills are also known as **oral hypoglycemic drugs**.

To learn more about oral diabetes medicine, visit:

ON THE WEB

http://effectivehealthcare.ahrq. gov/index.cfm/search-for-guides-reviews-and-reports/?productid=645&pageac tion=displayproduct

40. What is metformin, and how does it work?

Metformin belongs to a class of drugs called biguanides. It has various important actions, including:

- It reduces the amount of sugar that the body takes from food
- It reduces how much sugar the liver makes
- It helps the body respond better to insulin

For more information on metformin, visit:

ON THE WEB

http://www.nlm.nih.gov/medlineplus/druginfo/meds/a696005.html

Depending on the individual patient's situation, metformin can be used alone, or in combination with other drugs, including insulin.

41. I've heard of sulfonylurea drugs. What are they, and how do they work?

Sulfonylureas are also used to help reduce blood sugar levels. They are the first type of drug given to patients with type 2 diabetes who are not overweight and need to take pills. They work by helping:

- Beta cells in the pancreas to make more insulin
- The body to use insulin more efficiently

These include drugs like glyburide and glimepiride. Depending on the individual patient's situation, they can be used alone, or in combination with other drugs. In some studies, sulfonylureas have reduced HbA1c levels by 1% to 2%.

42. What is pioglitazone, and how does it work?

Pioglitazone belongs to a class of drugs called thiazolidinediones. It works by:

- Helping the body to use insulin more efficiently
- Reducing how much sugar the liver makes
- Saving the function of the beta cells in the pancreas

PRACTICAL TIP

If you need to take more than one of these drugs to help control your blood sugar, speak to your doctor about taking combination drugs. These are mixtures of two types of drugs. Combination drugs can be beneficial because they are cheaper than buying the two drugs separately, and they also reduce the number of pills you have to remember to take each day, making it easier to stick to your treatment plan.

Depending on the individual patient's situation, pioglitazone can be used alone, or in combination with other drugs.

Numerous other pills may be used to help lower blood sugar levels in patients with type 2 diabetes. These include:

Meglitinides: These help the pancreas to make more insulin after a meal. **Repaglinide** belongs to this class of drugs.

Incretin-based drugs: There are two types of these drugs.

- **DPP-4 inhibitors:** These slow the absorption of sugars into the blood after a meal. They also stop the release of glucagon, the other hormone made in the pancreas. Because glucagon works against insulin, this further reduces blood sugar levels. **Sitagliptin** belongs to this type.
- **GLP-1 analogs:** These help the pancreas to release enough insulin when blood sugar is high. Liraglutide belongs to this type.

Alpha-glucosidase inhibitors: These stop the action of an enzyme in the gut that usually helps break down carbohydrates in the diet. This delays the absorption of sugar from the gut, reducing the high swings of blood sugar after a meal. **Acarbose** belongs to this class of drugs.

Dapaglifozin: This belongs to a new class of drugs that cause sugar to be passed out in the urine. Dapaglifozin works

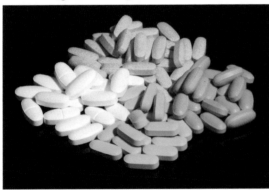

on the kidneys to stop the action of a transport mechanism that usually returns sugar to the blood as it passes through the kidneys. The sugar therefore passes out through the kidneys into the urine.

If you have type 2 diabetes and need help controlling your blood sugar levels, your doctor will choose an oral hypoglycemic drug that best suits your individual situation. This will take into account factors like your age, body weight, and whether you have liver, kidney, or heart disease.

Metformin is usually the first drug given to overweight patients with type 2 diabetes who need pills, because it does not cause weight gain. Sulfonylureas are typically the first type of drug given to patients with type 2 diabetes who are not overweight and need to take pills. They are also given to patients who cannot take metformin. Sulfonylureas may also cause low blood sugar, and therefore may not be the best choice of drug for elderly patients or those living alone.

In patients with kidney disease, drugs such as metformin and sitagliptin should be avoided. Liraglutide and insulin, however, are relatively safe for patients with kidney disease. Metformin and acarbose should not be used in patients with severe liver disease. Sulfonylureas seem to be safe in patients with liver disease. Thiazolidinediones such as pioglitazone may increase the risk of congestive heart failure (CHF) in patients who are at risk for this condition. Metformin should be avoided in patients with unstable CHF or those who are hospitalized with CHF.

 If traveling by airplane, keep your medications in your carry-on luggage. Make sure they are in their original containers with the pharmacy labels intact.

45. How do I monitor my glycemic control?

Glycemic control is another way of saying blood sugar control. Just as in type 1 diabetes, people with type 2 diabetes must monitor their blood sugar levels to keep them in a healthy range. The goal of treatment for type 2 diabetes is to keep blood sugar levels as close to normal as possible, to reduce the risk of complications of the disease. Your diabetes specialist will work with you to determine how you should monitor your blood sugar levels.

Self-monitoring with a blood sugar meter: This is commonly done at home if you have type 2 diabetes and need insulin. The frequency of testing will depend on what drugs you are taking to control your diabetes, and may be up to 3 or 4 times a day, or more. Experts advise aiming to keep your blood sugar levels between 70 and 130 mg/dL before meals, and less than 180 mg/dL 1 to 2 hours after meals. See Chapter 9 for more information on monitoring blood sugar levels.

If you are not taking insulin, you may not need to monitor your sugar levels at home. Your diabetes specialist will be able to advise you depending on your individual situation.

▼ FIGURE 10.1
HbA1c levels and blood sugar control.

HbA1c

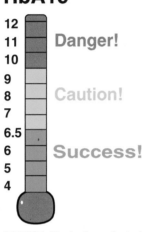

SOURCE: Illustration adapted from www.inspiredhygiene.com

HbA1c: HbA1c testing helps give you a picture of your overall blood sugar control during the past 3 months. The higher the HbA1c value, the poorer your blood sugar control.

If you have type 2 diabetes, the frequency of HbA1c testing will depend on how well your blood sugar is controlled. If you don't use insulin and your blood sugar is usually in a healthy range, you should have it tested twice a year. But if you use insulin and your blood sugar is difficult to keep in a healthy range, testing is advised four times each year to monitor how well your blood sugar is controlled. See Chapter 9 for more information on HbA1c.

To learn more about exams and tests in people with type 2 diabetes, visit:

ON THE WEB

http://www.nlm.nih.gov/medlineplus/ency/article/000313.htm

46. If I'm taking pills, do I still need to exercise and eat a healthy diet?

If you have been diagnosed with type 2 diabetes and need to take pills, exercise and diet are still very important parts of your treatment plan. (See Chapters 1, 17, and 18 for more details on exercise and healthy eating.)

For more information about the benefits of diet and exercise in people with type 2 diabetes, visit:

ON THE WEB

http://www.nlm.nih.gov/medlineplus/ency/article/007429.htm

Exercise will help you keep a healthy weight and prevent worsening of your condition, and will help control your blood pressure and cholesterol levels.

Physical activity will also boost your energy levels and your ability to burn calories, and these will help you lose weight. Regular exercise and a healthy diet may even help reduce the need for anti-diabetic pills in some people.

Insulin Therapy

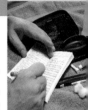

47. How do I know if I need insulin therapy?

Type 1 diabetes

If you have type 1 diabetes, because your pancreas no longer makes insulin, you will need to take insulin for life. Insulin is currently the only form of treatment available to control blood sugar levels in this type of the disease. Insulin therapy is typically started as soon as a diagnosis of type 1 diabetes is made. Since the condition can start suddenly, some people may need to stay in the hospital while insulin therapy is started, especially if symptoms are severe. Other patients can begin their insulin therapy at home, with regular follow-up visits to their doctor. Usually these visits will occur frequently until blood sugar levels are stabilized and your doctor feels your diabetes is under control and you are coping well with managing the disease. At this point, your follow-up visits will be less frequent, although you will still need to visit your doctor or diabetes healthcare professional in order to keep a check on how well your blood sugar is being controlled.

Type 2 diabetes

If you have type 2 diabetes, however, you may not need insulin therapy when you are first diagnosed. Because the body is resistant to insulin in patients with type 2 diabetes, eventually, over the course of time, the beta cells in the pancreas try to compensate for this by making more and more insulin. Eventually the cells may become exhausted and no longer able to make any insulin. This means that most people with type 2 diabetes will need insulin therapy eventually. The aim of providing insulin therapy is to mimic what the healthy pancreas is doing. Your need for insulin will depend on your blood sugar level, how long you have had the condition, your overall health, and what other drugs you are taking. And the decision to start insulin also depends on whether the patient is willing to try it.

There is no easy way to know when a patient with this type of the disease will benefit from insulin but there are some guidelines to help doctors decide when to start insulin therapy in these patients. Although doctors will determine what HbA1c level a patient should aim for if they have type 2 diabetes, some patients have trouble reaching this level with a combination of diet, exercise, and other drugs. In these situations, insulin therapy is advised in the short-term or long-term.

For information about when to start insulin therapy in patients with type 2 diabetes, see Document 11.1.InsTx

ON THE DVD

http://www.ccjm.org/content/78/5/332.long

48. What are the pros and cons of insulin therapy?

Patients with type 1 diabetes have no choice but to take insulin. Their pancreas is not producing any insulin, and because this hormone is needed to survive, it needs to be replaced.

Many patients with type 2 diabetes dread having to start taking insulin, and wait as long as possible before starting insulin therapy. As with any drug, there are pros and cons to starting insulin therapy (see Table 11.1).

Table 11.1 Pros and cons of insulin therapy in patients with type 2 diabetes

PROS	CONS
Insulin is the strongest drug available to control blood sugar levels	Insulin therapy causes weight gain, and this can be a problem especially in patients who are already overweight
Insulin is the most cost-effective drug for managing type 2 diabetes	Insulin increases the risk of low blood sugar levels which can be serious and fatal if they are too low
Insulin therapy lowers the risk of, or delays, the long-term complications of diabetes, such as blindness, heart attack, and stroke	Patients need to be trained to use insulin and require frequent visits to the doctor

Table 11.1 Continued

PROS	CONS
Many people who start insulin therapy report that it makes them feel better than they did before the therapy started	Some patients do not carry out the therapy effectively
	Some people are concerned about the pain of insulin injections
	Insulin therapy is a regimented process and interferes with daily life

But most patients with type 2 diabetes will have to take insulin eventually, and there is more and more evidence that starting insulin therapy earlier is better than waiting until there are no other options to try.

49. What are the different types of insulin?

There are 4 main types of insulin available (see Table 11.2):

- Fast-acting
- Regular-acting
- Intermediate acting
- Long-acting

These are classified based on:

- How quickly they begin to work after being injected
- How long they take to reach their maximum effect
- How long their effect lasts
- How they are given

Your doctor will help you decide which type of insulin is best for you. This will depend on factors such as:

- What type of diabetes you have
- How much your blood sugar changes throughout the day
- Your lifestyle

Your doctor may even give you different forms of insulin to use at different times of the day.

Table 11.2 The different types of insulin

FAST-ACTING	REGULAR-ACTING	INTERMEDIATE-ACTING	SLOW-ACTING
Begins to work within 15 minutes, and its effects last for up to 4 hours	Begins to work within 30 minutes, and its effects last for 3 to 6 hours	Begins to work within 2 to 4 hours, and its effects last for up to 18 hours	Begins to work within several hours, and works evenly throughout the day
Used to control blood sugar during meals, and to regulate high blood sugar		Used to control blood sugar overnight, during fasting, and in between meals	Used to control blood sugar overnight, during fasting, and in between meals

Pre-mixed insulin can also be helpful for some people who find it hard to use insulin from two different bottles and get the dosages right. This simplifies the insulin treatment plan, and is often used for people who are just starting to use insulin. It is also helpful for patients who don't see very well or have trouble using their hands, as well as older patients who have regular meal and activity schedules.

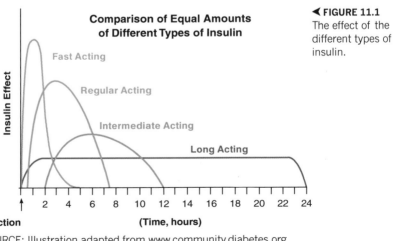

Comparison of Equal Amounts of Different Types of Insulin

◄ **FIGURE 11.1** The effect of the different types of insulin.

SOURCE: Illustration adapted from www.community.diabetes.org

Storing insulin

Your insulin supply—whether in the form of a bottle, cartridge, or pen—needs to be stored correctly, or it may not work effectively.

How you store insulin will depend on when you are going to use it:

- The insulin container you are using at the moment is best kept at room temperature (between 56°F and 80°F). Insulin is stable and works at its maximum ability for at least 28 days at room temperature. It is also more comfortable to inject.
- Keep unused insulin in the refrigerator (between 36°F and 46°F) and they will be good until the expiration date on the container.
- Keep your insulin away from heat and light because these will reduce its strength.
- Do not let your insulin freeze. If this happens, do not use the insulin even after it thaws, but discard it.
- When storing pre-filled insulin syringes, keep them with the needle pointing up.

Some helpful hints about your insulin supply:

- Write the start date on your insulin container so you will know when it needs to be thrown away.
- Never use insulin that has gone beyond its expiration date.
- Always keep extra insulin available at home in case of problems with your current supply.
- When traveling, keep your insulin in an insulated bag (like a lunch bag) and carry it with you.
- When traveling by plane, take your insulin in its original container with the prescription label. It can also be helpful to take a note from your pharmacist or doctor to say that you need to carry diabetes drugs and supplies.

ON THE WEB

For more information on how to store your insulin, visit:

http://www.youtube.com/watch?v=BctBQdY6zn8

For information on what to do with your insulin in the event of a prolonged power outage, visit:

http://www.youtube.com/watch?v=2YPo7g5cR1s

Insulin administration

There are 2 ways to deliver insulin (see Table 11.3):

- Injection
- Infusion

Table 11.3 How insulin is delivered

	INJECTION	INFUSION
INSULIN SYRINGE:	• The most common method used • Special insulin syringes are used • Insulin is injected into the fat under the skin	Infusion involves direct administration of insulin into a vein. This is sometimes needed when a patient is in hospital for surgery or in intensive care, for example. It is only done under medical supervision.
INSULIN PEN:	• It contains a replaceable cartridge that holds the insulin • It uses a replaceable needle • Has a dial to choose your insulin dose • Insulin is injected into the fat under the skin • Useful for active patients who need multiple injections, or people who don't see very well, or have trouble using their hands	
INSULIN PUMP:	• Small computerized device • Contains a pump, insulin reservoir, tubing, and infusion set • Insulin is injected into the fat under the skin	

Insulin is most commonly delivered by injection.

ON THE WEB

For more information on how to inject your insulin, visit:

http://www.youtube.com/watch?v=7-cGz2eLyb4

51. What are insulin pumps?

Insulin pumps are the most sophisticated devices used to deliver insulin, and are becoming more and more popular. They are especially useful because they continually deliver insulin and can therefore mimic how the healthy pancreas would produce insulin. They deliver exact doses of fast-acting insulin to match the body's needs, and this helps to improve blood sugar control. They can be set at a basal rate, involving small amounts being delivered continuously for the body's daily functions (not including food), or to give a bolus dose of insulin on-demand, such as at meal-times or if you need to correct your blood sugar level.

Insulin pumps consist of a:

- Pump reservoir to hold the insulin
- Battery-operated pump
- Computer chip that allows the patient to control how much insulin is being delivered
- Infusion set

▼ FIGURE 11.2
An insulin pump attached to the body via the infusion set.

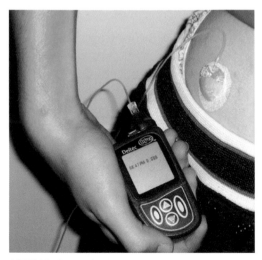

SOURCE: Commons Wikimedia

The pump is used for continuous delivery of insulin, and is attached to the infusion set—this is a plastic tube with a plastic needle called a cannula on the end. The cannula is placed under the skin and can be changed every 2 days.

Insulin pumps are small and can be attached to a belt, hidden under clothes, or kept in a pocket.

The plastic tube can be disconnected from the pump when the patient showers.

Many people prefer the insulin pump because they allow for tighter control of blood sugar, with fewer long-term diabetes complications. They also reduce the number of injections that are needed. Because they use fast-acting insulin, which is more predictable than long-acting insulin in how quickly it works, it helps you deliver small, precise doses of insulin whenever they are needed, and this prevents highs and lows of blood sugar.

52. How do I monitor my blood sugar levels while taking insulin?

Because of the complications of diabetes, it is important for patients to always be aware of their blood sugar levels.

Many of the newer insulin pumps have built-in sugar monitors, allowing for continuous monitoring of sugar levels, allowing for more accurate insulin delivery and better control of blood sugar. However, if you use one of the older pumps, or use insulin injections or an insulin pen, you will need to check your blood sugar levels yourself so that you know how much insulin you need.

In order to monitor your blood sugar levels effectively, you will need to know:

- **Your target blood sugar level:** Your doctor will help you determine what this is, and it may change during the course of your disease.
- **When to check your blood sugar:** Your doctor will tell you how often to check this. It may be multiple times each day, or just a few times each week, depending on your situation. But typical times are before breakfast, lunch, dinner, and bedtime. You may also need to check more frequently if you are sick, stressed, taking new medicines, pregnant, making changes to your treatment plan, or if you suspect that your blood sugar level is high or low.

To test your blood sugar level, you will use a device called a glucometer (glucose meter). Your doctor will help you choose which type is best for you, how to use it, and how to record the results.

The testing procedure is simple and quick. You will need:

- A glucometer
- Lancing device
- Test strip

ON THE WEB

For a video tutorial on how to test your blood sugar level, visit:

http://www.youtube.com/watch?v=wYprmjDuDwM

Here are the typical steps to follow:

1. Wash your hands

2. Clean your finger, or whatever site you are using to collect blood from, with alcohol

3. Prick the skin using a lancing device

4. Place a drop of blood on the test strip

5. Follow the instructions for using the test strip in the glucometer—some newer ones need you to place the strip into the meter before adding the blood, while older ones need the blood to be added to the strip before placing it into the meter

6. Check the blood sugar level recorded on the screen

7. Record the level

It can be helpful not to use the same finger or area of skin all the time, otherwise it can become painful. It may be helpful to use a different finger or region of skin each time you take your blood sample during a particular day.

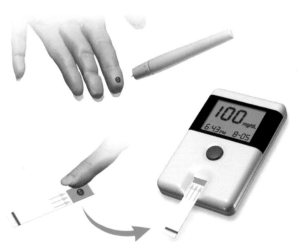

◀ FIGURE 11.3
Checking Your Blood Sugar Level Using a Glucometer.

SOURCE: Commons Wikimedia.

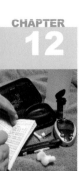

Other Drugs You Might Need, Including Those to Control Blood Pressure and Cholesterol Levels

53. Will I need to take drugs to lower my blood pressure?

Why is high blood pressure (BP) a problem?

When BP is too high (hypertension), the pressure is increased across all the systems of the body. The heart must therefore work harder to deliver blood throughout the body, and this increases the risk of heart disease and stroke.

Because diabetes leads to damage of the body's arteries and can contribute to them becoming hardened (atherosclerosis), it makes patients with diabetes more likely to develop high BP. This results in, and worsens, complications of diabetes such as kidney disease and eye disease if it is not treated properly.

What level of BP is too high?

In patients with diabetes, BP is considered high if it is higher than 130/80 mm Hg. And while lifestyle changes such as healthy eating (maintaining a good weight, not smoking, and reducing salt, alcohol, and caffeine intake, for example) and exercise are important to help control BP, most patients will also need drugs. About two in every three people with diabetes either have high (BP) or take drugs to lower their BP.

Exercise is an important part of a healthy lifestyle for patients with diabetes, especially to help manage high BP. If you are just starting out exercising, it is important to seek medical advice first. But as little as 30 minutes of moderate activity on most days of the week can be helpful—even if you need to break up your activity into three 10-minute sessions throughout the day.

PRACTICAL TIP

There are many types of drugs to treat high BP, and treatment selection is geared to each individual patient. Some patients may only need one drug to control their BP, but the American College of Cardiology and the

American Heart Association now recommend a combination of two or more drugs for people with BP above 140/90 mm Hg.

In most cases, high BP is symptomless. But because it can be very damaging to the body, and because it is commonly a problem in patients with diabetes, your doctor or other diabetes care specialists will carefully monitor your BP.

The decision to start or change BP treatment is not based on a single BP reading, because measurements can change throughout the day and in different environments. Your doctor will take multiple BP readings to get the best estimate of your true BP—this may include readings in your home, as well as in the doctor's office.

 For more information on how high BP increases the risk of kidney disease, and tips on keeping your kidneys healthy, visit:

http://www.cdc.gov/features/worldkidneyday/

What are some of the types of drugs available to treat high BP?

- **Angiotensin-converting enzyme (ACE) inhibitors**: Among the most commonly used type of drugs to treat high BP. Many doctors use ACE inhibitors first, and then add other types of drugs as necessary. These allow blood vessels to become wider by preventing formation of a hormone called angiotensin.
- **Diuretics (water pills)**: These work by flushing excess water and salt (sodium) from the body.
- **Angiotensin II receptor blockers**: These help blood vessels relax by blocking the action of angiotensin.
- **Beta blockers**: These work by blocking hormonal signals to the heart.
- **Calcium channel blockers**: These reduce BP by blocking calcium from getting into cells in the heart and blood vessels, allowing them to relax.
- **Renin inhibitors**: These work by reducing production of renin, and enzyme that is involved in increasing BP.

When it comes to preventing diabetes complications, managing your BP is as important as managing your blood sugar levels.

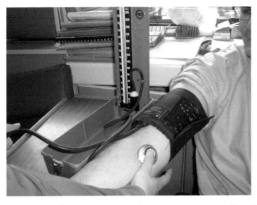

Why is high cholesterol a problem?

People with diabetes often have unhealthy cholesterol levels, and this can raise the risk for heart attack or stroke. The term "unhealthy cholesterol levels" refers to:

- Increased levels of low-density lipoprotein (LDL)—the so-called "bad cholesterol"
- Decreased levels of high-density lipoprotein (HDL)—the so-called "good cholesterol"
- Increased levels of triglycerides—fats in the body

For more information on cholesterol and triglycerides, visit:

http://diabetes.niddk.nih.gov/dm/pubs/complications_control/#should

ON THE WEB

Heart disease is the number one killer of patients with diabetes. Adults with diabetes are up to four times more at risk of developing heart disease or stroke than those who do not have diabetes.

So it is therefore especially important for patients with diabetes to take steps to reach healthy target levels of cholesterol and triglycerides.

Table 12.1 Ideal target blood levels in patients with diabetes

LDL cholesterol (mg/dL)	Less than 100
HDL cholesterol (mg/dL)	Men: more than 40 Women: more than 50
Triglycerides (mg/dL)	Less than 150

What drugs can help lower cholesterol?

There are various types of drugs available to help lower cholesterol levels, and your doctor will select which one—or combination—is best for you. However, statins are a commonly used type of cholesterol-lowering drug. They work by blocking a substance needed by the body to make cholesterol. They may also help the body to reabsorb cholesterol that has built up in plaques on the walls of arteries, stopping additional blockages in the blood vessels, and therefore helping to prevent heart attacks. Statin treatment usually continues long-term, even after your target cholesterol level is reached—this allows you to maintain the healthy level for as long as possible.

Just like the situation with high BP, lifestyle change is also important for reducing cholesterol to healthy levels, even if you are taking drugs such as a statin.

Because you are more likely to get heart disease if you have diabetes, your doctor or other diabetes care specialists will carefully monitor your cholesterol and triglyceride levels at least once a year.

PRACTICAL TIP Lifestyle changes can help reduce your risk of heart disease. You should keep a healthy weight—eating a heart-healthy diet is important for this—your diet should be low in fat, cholesterol, and salt. Exercising 30 minutes each day on most days of the week is helpful. Reduce how much alcohol you drink, and if you smoke, you should take steps to stop.

Managing Diabetes in Special Circumstances, Including Pregnancy, Childhood, and Others

55. I'm diabetic and I just found out I'm pregnant. What do I need to know about managing my diabetes?

Why is pregnancy a time of concern for women with diabetes?

Although most women with type 1 or type 2 diabetes have healthy pregnancies, the condition needs careful management during this time. Because of the hormonal changes during pregnancy, blood sugar levels rise during the first 4 to 6 weeks

To learn more about preparing for, and managing, pregnancy if you have diabetes, visit:

ON THE WEB

http://www.diabetes.niddk.nih.gov/dm/pubs/pregnancy/

and http://www.cdc.gov/features/diabetesandpregnancy/

in particular (see Figure 13.1). This increases the risk of having a baby with a birth defect to up to 40% if sugar levels are not controlled, compared with only 2% in women who do keep their diabetes well under control.

In addition to having a baby with a birth defect, women with type 1 or type 2 diabetes also have a higher risk of:

- Having a large baby: this increases the chance of needing a Caesarian delivery and complications during birth
- Stillbirth or miscarriage
- Premature birth
- **Pre-eclampsia**: a dangerous rise in blood pressure associated with protein in the urine
- Severe hypoglycemia
- **Diabetic kidney disease**
- **Diabetic eye disease** (retinopathy)

Because of the extra demands on a woman's body during pregnancy, it is important to carefully monitor your diabetes during this time, and make sure your sugar levels are kept under excellent control.

How should I monitor my diabetes now that I am pregnant?

If you are pregnant and have type 1 or type 2 diabetes, you should:

- Visit your doctor or diabetes specialist regularly (every 1 to 4 weeks, as needed)
- See a registered dietitian for help with your diet
- Have your HbA1c levels checked regularly (every 4 to 8 weeks)
- Exercise appropriately (ask your doctor for advice on how much exercise you need)
- Check your blood sugar before you drive
- Monitor your blood sugar levels frequently, especially before and after every meal

The American College of Obstetricians and Gynecologists (ACOG) recommend that blood sugar levels should be higher than 70 mg/dL, with upper limits varying depending on the time of day.

Table 13.1 ACOG recommendations for blood sugar levels during pregnancy

	BLOOD SUGAR LEVEL (Mg/dL)
Before meals	70–95
1 hour after eating	70–130
2 hours after eating	70–120

56. Are there any special strategies for managing gestational diabetes?

Gestational diabetes can be harmful to you and your baby, so it is important to get treatment quickly. But although this condition can be serious, women who manage it well can have successful pregnancies and healthy babies. Treatment aims to keep your blood sugar at similar levels to those of pregnant women who do not have gestational diabetes, as shown above in Table 13.1.

Some things you can do to help manage your gestational diabetes well:

- **Visit your doctor and obstetrician:** You will need to visit more often than women who do not have gestational diabetes. Ask if their office has a healthcare professional who specializes in high-risk pregnancies or diabetes. Your healthcare team will be able to monitor your condition throughout your pregnancy so that your treatment can be changed as necessary.
- **Visit a registered dietitian:** Because diet is the first line of treatment for gestational diabetes, you will need to pay even more attention to what you eat during pregnancy if you have this condition. Eating a healthy diet is important, and you should seek expert help to create a plan for this. A registered dietitian (RD) is an excellent choice for this—they will assess your diet and help you create meal plans to ensure your blood sugar stays in the required range. They will calculate the

amount of carbohydrates that you need at meals and for snacks, teach you how to count carbohydrates, and show you how to keep a food record. If you do not know where to find an RD, speak with your doctor, obstetrician, or a diabetes healthcare provider for advice on finding one, or for help with your diet. Although your dietary advice will be individual for you, there are some general recommendations that you may find helpful:

- Divide your daily food between 3 meals and 2 or 3 snacks per day.
- Although you need carbohydrates in your diet, be sure to eat only a reasonable portion (for example, 2 slices of bread, or 1 cup of total starch).
- Breakfast is important. Natural hormonal changes can make blood sugar control difficult in the morning. At this time, a breakfast of starch and protein tends to be tolerated best.
- Go easy on desserts and sweet things. This includes regular sodas and sugar-sweetened drinks. These all contain large amounts of carbohydrates.
- Watch your milk intake. Milk is a good calcium source, but it is also a form of carbohydrate and needs to be limited to approximately 1 cup at any time.
- Watch your fruit intake. Fruits are healthy, but they also contain carbohydrates and should be limited to 1 to 3 portions each day. A portion is either one small piece of fruit, half a large piece of fruit, or half a cup of mixed fruit. Canned fruit in syrup should be avoided. Fruit juice should also be avoided.

- Get regular, moderate exercise: even pregnant women with gestational diabetes should exercise, providing there is no health reason to prevent this. You should speak to your doctor or obstetrician before starting any exercise regime, but as little as 30 minutes of moderate activity on most days of the week can be helpful—even if you need to break up your activity into three 10-minute sessions throughout the day.
- Daily glucose testing and insulin injections may be needed: your doctor or obstetrician will determine whether you need insulin therapy while you are pregnant. If you do need insulin, you will be taught how

to administer it and change your dose as needed. You will also be taught how and when to monitor your blood sugar levels so you know how much insulin you need.

After pregnancy, the symptoms of diabetes typically disappear in women who with gestational diabetes. Your doctor or obstetrician will monitor you during your office visits following the birth to make sure your blood sugar levels have returned to normal. A small number of women continue to have diabetes after they give birth, so it is important for your healthcare provider to check for this, in case you need ongoing diabetes care.

To learn more about managing gestational diabetes, visit:

https://www.nichd.nih.gov/ publications/pubs/gest_diabetes/ Pages/index.aspx

▼ FIGURE 13.1
The relationship between pregnancy hormones and gestational diabetes.

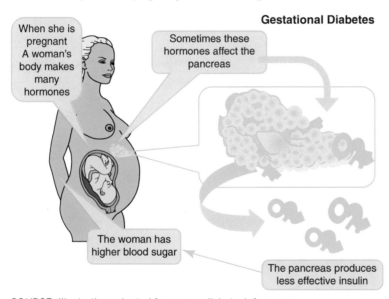

SOURCE: Illustration adapted from www.diabetesinfo.org.au

57. I have a child with diabetes. What are some strategies that might help me manage their condition effectively?

Although diabetes is a serious condition, if managed well, children with this condition are able to live long, healthy lives. If you have a child with diabetes, here are some tips to make it easier for you to help them manage their condition:

- *Be honest and patient with your child.* It is important to be direct with them about their condition. Avoid speaking to them about diabetes in a way that either minimizes the condition or dramatizes it. How you react to it will determine how they react.
- *Maintain control over their diabetes care, without smothering them.* Even older children need guidance, no matter how independent they are. So children of all ages should be monitored to some degree—the extent of this supervision will depend on their age and how well you observe them managing their condition over time. Help them set up a blood sugar and/or food diary, and check it with them.
- *Encourage your child to be central in the management of their diabetes.* Improvements in design of blood sugar meters and insulin pens and pumps have made it easier for children to use, either alone or with supervision—even many children of grade-school age.
- *Let them speak to a diabetes healthcare specialist regularly.* They may be more willing to talk openly about their condition, problems they are having managing it, and how they feel about it in general, with someone who isn't a family member. Speaking to a diabetes healthcare professional regularly—at least 4 times per year—will therefore enable any problems to be identified and addressed more quickly than if you are relying on them talking to you or another family member.
- *Make it a family affair.* Instead of creating special meals and exercise plans for your child with diabetes, get everyone in the family on the same level. Feed everyone the same healthy diet, consisting of low-fat, whole grains, fresh fruits, and vegetables. And have everyone involved in the same exercise activities—at least 60 minutes of exercise should be encouraged each day, unless their doctor suggests otherwise.
- *Don't hold them back.* Just because they have diabetes, this doesn't mean they can't strive for things that interest them. If your child wants to play college football, or train for a marathon, don't make them fearful of their condition. If they have the physical ability to achieve their sporting dream, for instance, so long as they

manage their diabetes well and their doctor has given the go-ahead for them to train, there is no reason why they should not participate in competition sports.

- *Communicate with their school.* You can't be with your child every minute of the day to monitor their condition. And even though they will hopefully be very independent and capable of managing their diabetes effectively, it is always a good idea to make sure you can connect with someone responsible at their school who can help them during the school day. This may be a teacher or a school nurse—someone who is trained to deal with children who have diabetes, whether to help them check blood sugar levels, or recognize and manage the signs and symptoms of hypoglycemia. The same principle applies to other situations, such as group trips or visits to friends' houses. Make sure a responsible adult is always available to help your child with his or her diabetes care needs—someone who is willing to take on this role as and when necessary, and is able to deal with any potential emergency situation.

For information on helping your child manage diabetes at school, visit:

http://www.cdc.gov/features/diabetesinschool/

- *Make sure your child has access to the necessary diabetes supplies.* You can put together a pack for your child to take in their bag to school, on trips, or when visiting friends. This will contain all the items they need to manage their diabetes.

Importantly, your child should not identify him- or herself by their diabetes. Although it is essential for them to manage their condition well, and for you to be active in supervising this, diabetes should not be all that you talk about when your child comes home from school, for example. Talk with them about their day, just as you would do if they did not have diabetes. Their diabetes is a part of their life—not all of it.

When creating a diabetes care pack for your child, some important things to think about including are: insulin supply (including a backup supply, as necessary); blood sugar test strips and a lancet; blood sugar meter and spare batteries; blood sugar record book or record sheets; fast-acting sugar snacks (glucose tablets or hard candy).

The issues facing seniors with diabetes are similar in those with the type 1 and type 2 forms of the condition. Serious diabetes complications such as problems with hearing, eyesight, kidney function, mobility, heart disease, stroke, and cognitive (mental) functioning are particularly troublesome for older people. This is true even for people who do control their diabetes well, not just those who have problems controlling their blood sugar.

1 in 4 Americans 65 years or older have type 2 diabetes, and this number is expected to grow in the coming decades.

Prevention is key

One of the key things in managing older patients is prevention of diabetes complications. Although they may seem to be doing well with their diabetes control, often when something goes wrong, older patients can deteriorate quickly. So health assessments should be more frequent in older patients with diabetes than in younger ones. This allows the diabetes healthcare team to monitor the risk of the patient's complications, screen them for problems, and manage their care appropriately—and, importantly, on a level that is personalized for their specific needs.

Managing diabetes medicines

One important issue for older patients with diabetes is managing their medicines, especially to prevent side effects associated with their drugs. Many drugs can be hazardous for older patients, so it is critical that they are not taken for longer than necessary, and that patients are watched for side effects. If patients are being monitored by their doctor frequently, assessments of their medicines and reactions can therefore become an ongoing part of their diabetes care. Some complications are of particular concern in older patients with diabetes:

- Hypoglycemia is one of the most common diabetes medicine complications, especially in patients who are frail or have dementia. This can leave patients at increased risk for falls and therefore fractures, as well as cognitive problems. HbA1c levels should therefore be stabilized at around 8.5%. Anything less puts patients at high risk of hypoglycemia, and higher levels leave them at risk of hyperglycemia (high blood sugar).

- Hyperglycemia, on the other hand, leaves older patients at increased risk for urinary tract infections and foot wound infections. Foot infections are of concern because of the risk of the patient needing amputations, and at worst, some may even die from these infections. A hyperosmolar state can also arise in association with hyperglycemia, causing patients to become very dehydrated. This can also be a cause for concern because it can result in cognitive difficulties and delirium, and patients may even need to be hospitalized—up to a third may even die as a result of this problem.

The focus of diabetes care for older patients has increasingly become one of personalizing health care according to what is important for each individual patient, rather than merely on aggressive control of blood sugar levels. Older patients in good health might benefit from more aggressive diabetes control because they are likely to live longer and enjoy the rewards of strict sugar control. However, an older, frail patient in a nursing home who also has other medical conditions is less likely to benefit from strict blood sugar control. So looser goals might be better for some patients.

 For information on diabetes in older patients with kidney disease, see Document 13.1.DKid

http://www.revistanefrologia.com/revistas/P1-E569/P1-E569-S4583-A12319-EN.pdf

59. I have a hospital stay planned. How do I make sure my diabetes is properly managed?

If you have diabetes, no doubt you have developed your own daily routines and strategies to allow you to manage your diabetes well. Any change to your routine may result in problems, so being in hospital—whether for a planned procedure or a sudden illness—can therefore be a challenging time. This is especially true with regards to your diet.

Why is it important to control my blood sugar levels in hospital?

Diabetes puts patients at higher risk of complications in the hospital. These include harmful swings of blood sugar levels, falls, infections, and pressure ulcers. Very high blood sugar levels can slow the healing process and increase the risk of infection, while low sugar levels can increase the risk of falls and fractures. Excellent control of diabetes around the time of a surgery has been shown to reduce illness, duration of hospital stay, and even the risk of death.

If you have to stay in the hospital, your routine will be challenged in many ways, so it is especially important to take extra precautions to manage your blood sugar levels in hospital. Some challenges include:

- *A change in your medicine regime:* If you are having surgery, you may be taken off your sugar control medicines the night before. You may also need to fast and stop drinking fluids for a period of time beforehand. You will likely be scheduled for a planned surgery in the morning to reduce how long you have to stop your medicines, but it is a good idea to ask your surgeon about this.
- *A change in your physical activity level:* Your exercise level will be reduced while you are in hospital, whether due to forced bed rest, or simply not being able to perform your usual level of physical activities each day. This may drive up your blood sugar levels more than usual.
- *A change in your meals:* Loss of control over the timing of meals, as well as the types of foods and snacks you have access to, may increase the risk of hypoglycemia.
- *A change in target blood sugar levels:* The American Diabetes Association recommends a blood sugar range of 140–180 mg/dL for most critically ill hospital patients on insulin treatment, although more strict control may be required in some circumstances. While there is no clear evidence for goals in non-critically ill patients on insulin treatment, they recommend a pre-meal target of less than or equal to 140 mg/dL blood sugar, with random blood sugar readings of less than 180 mg/dL.

To learn more about diabetes care in various settings, including hospital stays, see Document 13.2.DHosp

http://care.diabetesjournals.org/content/37/Supplement_1/S14.full.pdf+html

Who will take control over my blood sugar levels while I am in the hospital?

Whether or not you can manage your own blood sugar levels in the hospital will depend on various things, such as your physical condition, the reason you are being hospitalized, and the hospital's policy. Speak to the hospital's diabetes care team to find out whether you can take control of your diabetes while you are there.

If you are able to do so, be sure to take along all the necessary diabetes items you will need during your stay. If your hospital stay is unplanned but you are still able to control your own diabetes, ask a family member or friend to bring you all the items you will need. It is helpful to have either a diabetes care pack ready and easily accessible at home in case someone needs to collect it in your absence—or at least a list of all the items you need, and detailed instructions on where they can be found.

During your stay, make sure there is somewhere in your ward where you can safely and appropriately store your insulin and other diabetes items. You must also record your insulin doses on your hospital chart, and make sure the hospital care team has access to your blood sugar results.

If you are unable to control your own blood sugar levels while in the hospital, speak to the team who will be in charge of doing this for you. Be sure to let them know your particular symptoms of low or high blood sugar, and any other specific needs you have.

PRACTICAL TIP Put together your diabetes care pack (or at least keep a list of all the items you might need someone to collect for you) so you are prepared for an emergency. Items you might need to have include: insulin supply (including a backup supply, as necessary); blood sugar test strips and a lancet; blood sugar meter and spare batteries; blood sugar record book or sheets; fast-acting sugar snacks (glucose tablets or hard candy).

What about my meal plan?

It is important to speak to the hospital dietitian about your dietary needs—especially if you have very specific needs with regard to the foods you eat, and when you have to eat them. If your hospital trip is a planned one, you can speak to the dietitian in advance so they have a record of your dietary needs and can plan for your meals.

During your stay, be sure to let someone know as soon as possible if you are given the wrong foods, or your meals don't arrive on time.

How can I make sure everyone knows about my diabetes?

Although your doctor will communicate to your hospital team that you have diabetes, it is always good to remind all of the healthcare professionals that care for you about your condition. Your diabetes status should also be recorded on your hospital in-patient chart, so you can also check on this. Additionally, make sure you are wearing some type of visible medical identification.

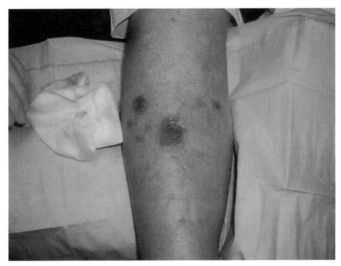

◀ FIGURE 13.2
Skin ulcer on the leg of a patient with diabetes.

SOURCE: Commons Wikimedia

So, although a hospital stay can be a particularly anxiety-provoking time for you if you have diabetes, the good news is that there are various things you can do to manage your condition effectively. This will help to maximize your diabetes care, and therefore reduce the duration of your hospital stay and allow for the best health outcome.

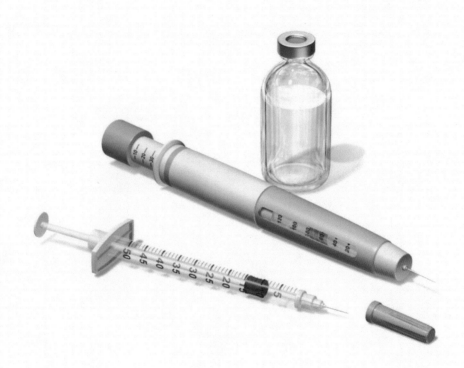

PART FIVE

Complications of Diabetes

In Part Five, we will discuss the progression of diabetes and its complications. We will take a look at the acute complications of diabetes, in particular hypoglycemia and ketoacidosis, as well as its long-term complications, such as blindness and kidney disease, addressing how to monitor for these diabetic complications during the course of the disease.

CHAPTER 14

Acute Complications of Diabetes, Including Hypoglycemia and Ketoacidosis

CHAPTER 15

Long-Term Complications of Diabetes, Including Blindness, Kidney Disease, and Others

Acute Complications of Diabetes, Including Hypoglycemia and Ketoacidosis

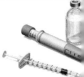

CHAPTER 14

60. What are the acute complications of diabetes?

There are several acute (short-term) complications of diabetes. These can be serious and life-threatening, and may arise quickly. Thankfully they can go away just as quickly if you know what to do when the situation arises.

Acute complications can affect numerous parts of the body, and arise from uncontrolled high (hyperglycemia) and low blood sugar levels (hypoglycemia) that result from having taken too little diabetes medicine or too much. Some acute complications require immediate medical attention, and these include hypoglycemia, a hyperosmolar state, and diabetic ketoacidosis.

61. What is hypoglycemia, and what commonly causes it?

Hypoglycemia (low blood sugar level) occurs when the brain and body do not receive enough sugar to provide energy for the body's activities.

For most people, a blood sugar level less than 70 mg/dl is considered low. Sometimes it's also difficult to know why this happens, but some things that can raise the odds of hypoglycemia occurring include:

- A delayed meal or snack.
- Not eating enough carbohydrates.
- Drinking a lot of alcohol, especially without food.
- Unplanned exercise.
- Taking too much insulin or other diabetes medicines such as insulin-releasing pills (sulfonylureas, meglitinides, or nateglinide). If you have type 2 diabetes, however, and are only treated with lifestyle changes or blood sugar

normalizing medicines, it is unlikely that you will suffer low blood sugar levels.

Symptoms

Hypoglycemia can come on quickly, causing different symptoms in different people, but some common ones are:

- Feeling shaky
- Hunger
- Sweating or chills
- Feeling tired or moody
- Blurry vision
- Headaches
- Confusion
- Lack of concentration
- Seizures

Treating hypogylcemia

Don't wait for your first episode of hypoglycemia to know how to deal with it. Make sure you (and your family, friends, co-workers, caretakers) are ready for it. If necessary, leave a note with instructions visible somewhere at home, and carry one on your person when you are out alone.

See how to recognize and deal with a hypoglycemic episode:

http://www.youtube.com/watch?v=K_Yh8_nFZIk

ON THE WEB

If you are conscious

- Treat your hypoglycemia immediately with 15–20g of fast-acting carbohydrate (see Practical Tip). Avoid foods that are high in fat (such as chocolate and cookies)—the fat will delay the absorption of the sugar, and won't treat the hypoglycemia quickly enough.
- Re-test your blood sugar levels after 15 to 20 minutes, and re-treat with fast-acting carbohydrate if your blood sugar levels are still too low.

15 to 20 grams of fast-acting carbohydrate

PRACTICAL TIP

- Candies such as jelly beans or hard candies (check the package to see how many you need to make up 15 grams of glucose)
- Glucose tablets (check the package to see how many you need)
- Glucose gel (check the package to see how much you need)
- Small glass of sugary (non-diet) drink
- Small carton of pure fruit juice
- One tablespoon of sugar or honey

- When your blood sugar has returned to normal, eat a small snack if your next planned meal is still an hour or two away.
- If necessary—for instance, if you feel like you are going to pass out and are alone or with people who are not sure how to help you, call 911 for assistance.

If you are unconscious

If untreated, hypoglycemia can cause you to pass out, have seizures, or go into a coma. In this case, someone else needs to take over immediate treatment—so it is critical that people you are in contact with know what to do if this severe situation arises.

They will need to administer glucagon to you, a hormone that helps the liver to release sugar when your blood sugar levels are too low. Make sure people know where to find your glucagon kit, and also make them aware in advance that if you should experience symptoms of severe hypoglycemia, they will need to:

- Call 911.
- Inject glucagon into your arm, thigh, or buttock, following instructions on the glucagon package.
- Be aware that it may take up to 15 minutes for you to become conscious again. At this time you may vomit or feel sick.

If you do need to use glucagon, let your doctor know as soon as possible so you can talk about how to prevent hypoglycemia happening in the future.

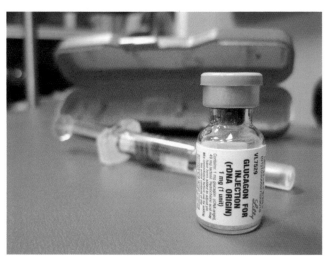

◄ FIGURE 14.1
Glucagon for injection.

SOURCE: Commons Wikimedia

A **hyperglycemic/hyperosmolar state (HHS)** is a life-threatening emergency situation. It arises in people who do not know they have diabetes, or those whose diabetes is not controlled properly, and it is often associated with something like illness or infection. These situations lead to blood sugar levels that are extremely high—more than 600 mg/dL. Although it is uncommon, it is life threatening. It can occur in people with type 1 or type 2 diabetes, but does occur more commonly in association with type 2, and is more frequently in older patients. It can take days or even weeks for HHS to develop.

HHS is a vicious cycle where high blood sugar levels cause you to urinate a lot and become dehydrated. This causes the blood to become more concentrated, leading to even higher blood sugar levels. The body now works even harder to get rid of the excess sugar in the urine, and this makes the dehydration worse. Ketone levels are usually normal or only slightly high.

Symptoms and signs

- Extreme thirst
- Dry mouth
- Warm skin that does not sweat
- Tiredness and confusion
- Loss of vision
- Frequent urination
- Later you will urinate less, and your urine may be dark
- High fever (more than 101 degrees Farenheit)
- Blood sugar over 600 mg/dL
- Seizures
- Coma

HHS usually happens to people who don't know they have diabetes. It also happens to people who know they have diabetes and are sick with something else and don't check their blood sugars or drink enough fluid.

For more information on the causes and symptoms of HHS, visit:

ON THE WEB

http://www.nlm.nih.gov/medlineplus/ency/article/000304.htm

Treatment

HHS is a serious complication—it is an emergency situation that can lead to death if not dealt with properly. Immediate hospitalization is necessary, and you may need to be treated with low-dose insulin and intravenous fluids.

It is a situation that is best avoided by controlling your diabetes properly, so it is very important to check your blood sugar levels regularly. If you are sick, make sure you check your blood sugar more frequently, and drink plenty of water.

63. What are the symptoms of diabetic ketoacidosis, and what causes it?

Diabetic Ketoacidosis (DKA) is a life-threatening emergency condition that arises when someone with diabetes does not get enough insulin, and leads to a diabetic coma or even death if not treated urgently. It is more common in patients with type 1 diabetes, but can occur on occasions in someone with type 2 diabetes if they get another serious medical condition, or are being treated with steroids.

For more information on the diagnosis and management of hyperglycemic emergencies, including HHS and diabetic ketoacidosis, see Document 14.1.Hyper

http://www.hormones.gr/pdf/HORMONES%202011-250-260.pdf

What causes DKA?

If you don't get enough insulin, your body's cells don't get enough sugar to feed their energy requirements. Your body therefore has to burn fat for energy. This process releases ketones—acids that build up in the bloodstream and then appear in the urine. Ketones are a sign that your diabetes is out of control or that you are getting sick.

A lack of insulin usually due to:

- Not enough insulin: This occurs in unknown or newly diagnosed cases of type 1 diabetes. It can occur in patients who take insulin and have missed a dose, not taken enough, or even used spoiled insulin. This may also be a problem in patients who are sick, especially those with a serious medical condition (like a severe infection or acute pancreatitis) who might need more insulin. Patients on steroid treatment may also need more insulin because steroids can cause insulin resistance.
- Not enough food: If you don't eat enough food, particularly if you are sick and have a poor appetite, this may cause you to have high ketone levels.

- Insulin reaction: If you have high ketone levels in the morning, this may be due to an insulin reaction occurring while you were asleep, resulting in low blood sugar levels.

Early symptoms

DKA typically develops slowly, and some of the early warning signs include:

- Feeling thirsty
- Dry mouth
- High blood sugar levels (although not always)

For more information on the causes and symptoms of DKA, visit:

ON THE WEB

http://www.nlm.nih.gov/medlineplus/ency/article/000320.htm

Later symptoms

- Vomiting—once vomiting occurs, a life-threatening situation can occur within a few hours
- Nausea
- Stomach pain
- Feeling thirsty
- Urinating a lot
- Fruity breath due to the smell of ketones
- Feeling tired or weak
- Speech problems, confusion, or unconsciousness
- Heavy, deep breathing

How can I check for ketones?

You can check for ketones by a simple urine test, using test strips similar to those used to check your blood sugar levels.

When should I check my urine for ketones?

Test your urine for ketones:

- If your blood sugar levels are higher than 250 mg/dL
- If you are sick
- If you are planning to exercise and your blood sugar is more than 250 mg/dL
- If you are pregnant, check for ketones every morning before breakfast

Treatment

If your urine contains ketones, call your doctor immediately, as you may need extra insulin. You should also:

- Drink plenty of water
- Check your blood sugar levels every 3 to 4 hours, and test for ketones any time the sugar level is more than 250 mg/dL
- Avoid exercise if your blood sugar level is high and you have ketones in your urine

Your doctor will determine whether you need urgent medical attention, which may include:

- Hospitalization
- Intravenous insulin treatment
- Intravenous fluids

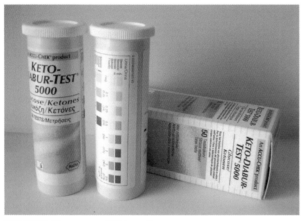

◄ **FIGURE 14.2**
Ketone test strips.

SOURCE: Commons Wikimedia

Long-Term Complications of Diabetes, Including Blindness, Kidney Disease, and Others

64. What are the risk factors for long-term complications?

Chronic (long-term) complications do not arise in every patient with diabetes, but when they do, they develop over years or even decades, so the symptoms may not be noticed. However, by the time symptoms are noticeable, the damage has already been done. Routine screening is therefore recommended to catch and treat long-term complications as soon as possible, and minimize damage to the body.

Common long-term diabetes complications can affect your:

- Eyes
- Kidneys
- Nerves
- Sexual function
- Feet
- Teeth and gums
- Heart

Certain things may increase the risk of developing long-term complications. These include:

- High blood sugar levels
- Smoking
- An unhealthy diet
- A sedentary lifestyle
- High blood pressure
- The length of time you have had diabetes
- Inheriting a genetic tendency for certain risk factors

Although some of these can be controlled (such as whether you smoke, and the kind of diet and lifestyle you choose), others cannot be controlled (such as your genetic risk, or how long you have had diabetes).

However, if any long-term complications do develop, controlling your blood sugar levels well can help slow down how quickly they progress.

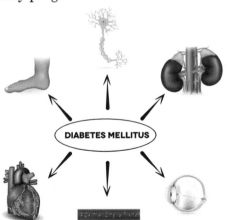

◀ **FIGURE 15.1**
Long-term effects of diabetes on the body.

SOURCE: Shutterstock

DIABETES MELLITUS

65. What is diabetic eye disease?

Diabetic eye disease is a leading cause of blindness, and refers to a group of eye problems that patients with diabetes may develop as a result of long-term complications of the disease. High blood sugar levels can damage the eyes over time, causing eye problems such as:

- Diabetic retinopathy, where the blood vessels at the back of the eye in the retina are damaged
- Cataract, where the lens of the eye is diseased
- Glaucoma, where a buildup of fluid in the eye increases the pressure inside the eye, leading to damage to the optic nerve and vision loss

ON THE WEB

To see how diabetes increases the risk of eye disease, visit:

http://nihseniorhealth.gov/diabeticretinopathy/whatisdiabeticretinopathy/video/dr1_na.html?intro=yes

However, a combination of regular screening with eye exams by your eye doctor, and keeping good control of your blood sugar levels can help to avoid most of these serious eye problems, or successfully treat them.

66. How does diabetes affect the kidney?

One job of the kidneys is to selectively filter waste products from the blood so that they can be removed from the body in the urine, while keeping useful substances in the blood. Over time, the high blood sugar levels of uncontrolled diabetes can make the kidneys work too hard at filtering the blood. Eventually, this extra work damages the kidney's filter system, and it starts to become leaky. This ultimately allows useful proteins to be lost through the kidney's filters into the urine (see Figure 15.2).

This damage to the kidneys in patients with diabetes is known as diabetic nephropathy. Early on, when only a small amount of protein is being lost in the urine, this is known as microalbuminuria, and treatment at this time can slow down the worsening of the condition. However, later, when larger amounts are lost, it is known as macroalbuminuria. If the kidney disease is not detected until this later time, end-stage renal disease (ESRD) usually follows. *ESRD* occurs when the kidneys *stop* working well enough for a patient to live without dialysis or a kidney *transplant*. This damage is permanent and cannot be fixed.

Since early diagnosis and treatment of kidney disease may successfully stabilize and maintain kidney function, it is important to visit a doctor regularly to check your blood pressure, and for routine screening using blood tests to check your kidney function by test for build-up of waste products in the bloodstream. This will help prevent ESRD.

Some things you can do to help prevent diabetic kidney disease include:

- Keep excellent control over your blood sugar levels. This can reduce the risk of developing microalbuminuria by one third, and if it is already present, can halve the risk of it progressing to macroalbuminuria.
- Manage your blood pressure at a healthy level.
- Keep your blood cholesterol levels at a healthy level.
- Not smoking.
- Avoid pain medicines that can hurt your kidneys (such as nonsteroidal anti-inflammatory drugs).
- Visit your doctor at least once a year for blood tests to check your kidney function, and urine tests to check for protein leakage.

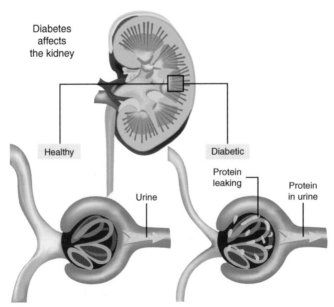

◄ FIGURE 15.2
How diabetes affects the kidney.

SOURCE: Illustration adapted from www.nation.lk

67. Does diabetes lead to nerve damage?

People with diabetes can get nerve damage, also known as diabetic neuropathy, if they have high blood sugar levels for a long time. This is because the high sugar levels can damage the protective covering and blood vessels around nerves, and may prevent the nerves doing their job of sending signals effectively throughout the body.

It usually affects the feet and toes first, but can progress up the legs, and even affect the hands. Although some people do not experience symptoms, when they do occur, they can include:

- Numbness
- Tingling
- Burning or shooting pains
- Feeling light touch as painful
- Urinary problems
- Problems with sexual function

Your doctor will check to see if you have diabetic neuropathy by giving you a physical exam and performing nerve tests.

Some things you can do to help protect your feet and prevent or manage nerve damage include:

- Keep excellent control over your blood sugar levels.
- Taking good care of your feet to either prevent problems, or prevent a mild problem becoming a more serious one.
- Visiting your doctor at least once a year for a complete foot examination, and having your doctor do a quick check of your feet each time you visit.

68. Can diabetes cause sexual problems?

Type 1 and type 2 diabetes can both cause sexual problems. As many as 50% of men and 25% of women may experience a loss of sexual desire or problems with sexual performance. Any swings in blood sugar levels can make you feel more tired in general, and this factor alone can lower your sexual desire.

In men, erectile dysfunction may result from the complications of diabetic nerve or blood vessel damage, or both. If this occurs in the erectile tissue of the penis, the man may have problems getting or keeping an erection. This is how some men eventually discover they have diabetes.

In women, the clitoris may not respond well to stimulation, for a similar reason that the man's penis is affected. Inflammation can also occur in the vagina (vaginitis), resulting in itching or burning. Vaginal dryness may also occur, making sex uncomfortable or painful.

To see how diabetes can affect sexual function, visit:

http://diabetes.niddk.nih.gov/dm/pubs/sup/

ON THE WEB

Hypoglycemia can also occur in men and women during sex, especially due to the physical activity involved. So you must be careful to test your sugar levels before and after, to prevent this happening.

Excellent management of diabetes through diet, exercise, and medication, however, can help to reduce problems that are relatively mild. Some cases may need more help though. For instance, some men with erectile dysfunction may need to try additional treatments to deal with erectile problems, such as using a vacuum pump or having injections into the penis. Some may even require surgery. Women may need to use vaginal lubricant, or to learn techniques to improve sexual response, like changes in position and stimulation during sex, as well as things such as Kegel exercises to help strengthen the pelvic muscles.

Speak to your healthcare provider if you have diabetes and experience any problems with sexual desire or performance, so that you can get the help you need managing your blood sugar levels, and additional treatments if necessary.

69. Does diabetes lead to foot disease?

In people with diabetes, foot problems may result from the complications of diabetic nerve or blood vessel damage, or both:

- Problems with sensation, such as pain or numbness
- Wounds may heal slowly
- Infections may be more common
- Joints may become deformed

The loss of sensation is a big problem because it means you may not realize you have blisters or cuts on your feet. It can also change the way you walk, or even damage the bones and joints. If your circulation is poor, this prevents adequate numbers of white blood cells from being able to get to the site of a wound quickly enough to fight infection, and reduces how effectively antibiotic medications in the blood can reach the affected area. Any delay in treatment can lead to serious problems, so you should see your doctor as soon as possible if you notice any foot problems.

PRACTICAL TIP There are many ways to protect your feet: always wear shoes or slippers; wear shoes and socks that fit well and are not too tight; change your socks daily; trim your toe nails carefully; wash your feet with soap and warm water daily and apply moisturizing lotion when dry; check your feet daily for signs of cuts, swellings, redness, blisters, and open sores, and seek medical attention if anything concerns you, or if sores do not go away. And last, but not least, control your blood glucose as well as possible.

70. Does diabetes increase my risk of dental problems?

Some people with diabetes can develop periodontal disease (infection and inflammation of the gums), because high blood sugar levels can cause gum inflammation and lead to bacterial and yeast infection in the mouth. Eventually the periodontal disease can lead to gum recession where the gum tissue around the tooth wears away over time, risking exposure of the tooth roots. Caries can also result.

Be sure to tell your dentist if you have diabetes, so he or she can advise you on how to keep your teeth and gums as healthy as possible. Visit your dentist and hygienist regularly, and follow their instructions for brushing and flossing your teeth. Finally, avoid smoking.

ON THE WEB To see how diabetes can affect your teeth, visit:

http://diabetes.niddk.nih.gov/dm/pubs/complications_teeth/

71. Does diabetes increase my risk of heart disease?

Diabetes and prediabetes both increase your risk of developing heart disease or stroke. Even mildly high blood sugar levels in people with prediabetes can increase the risk of heart disease. Vascular disease (disease of the blood vessels which can lead to stroke) is more common in people with diabetes, and is caused by atherosclerosis (stiffening and blocking of arteries). When blood sugar levels are constantly high over a long time, large amounts of fatty materials (plaque) stick to the inside walls of the blood vessels, making them harder and less stretchy. High blood sugars also contribute to atherosclerosis by leading to plaque formation. Certain traits and conditions like high blood pressure, high cholesterol and triglyceride levels, and smoking all further increase the risk of these problems occurring.

If you have diabetes, you are also at a higher risk of developing heart disease or stroke at a younger age than people who do not have diabetes. If you have diabetes and have already had one heart attack, you are at a higher risk of having another one. Heart attacks in people with diabetes are also more serious, with a higher chance of causing death. Heart disease may also be silent, so there may be no symptoms, even while a heart attack is occurring.

72. Will lowering my cholesterol levels help to reduce the risk of heart disease?

Lowering your cholesterol levels will definitely help lower your risk of heart disease. Diabetes tends to reduce "good" (high density lipoprotein—HDL) cholesterol levels and raise triglyceride and "bad" (low density lipoprotein—LDL) cholesterol levels. This combination raises the risk for heart disease and stroke.

To reduce this risk, some recommendations include:

- Making sure the total cholesterol (found in eggs, meat, and dairy products in particular) in your diet amounts to less than 300 mg per day.
- Having the majority of fats in your diet be monounsaturated or polyunsaturated.
- Lowering your saturated fat intake. The American Heart Association recommends making sure saturated fats in your diet do not total more than 5% to 6% of total calories (about 111 to 13 grams for someone eating 2,000 calories per day in their diet).

- Lowering how many calories in your diet come from *trans* fat. This type of fat can increase blood cholesterol. It is found in things like cookies, crackers, cake mixes, fried foods, and other foods made with partially hydrogenated oil. Avoid eating more than 1% of your daily calories as *trans* fat. This equals less than 20 grams of *trans* fats if you eat 2,000 calories in your diet each day.
- Eating at least 14 grams of fiber for every 1,000 calories in your diet. Foods high in fiber include things like whole-wheat bread, fruits, vegetables, oatmeal, and cereals.

Make an appointment with a registered dietitian to get help making a diet plan that will help lower your cholesterol levels and is generally heart-healthy.

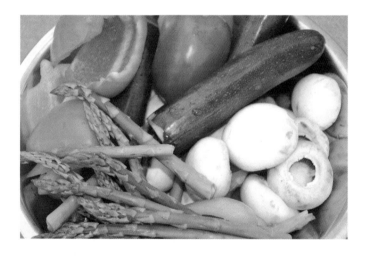

73. Does blood pressure management help to reduce the risk of heart disease?

Lowering your blood pressure will definitely help lower your risk of heart disease. High blood pressure (hypertension) is the most important risk factor for early heart disease. It accounts for approximately half of all strokes and heart attacks. The risk for coronary artery disease (atherosclerosis) and stroke continue to rise with stepwise increases in blood pressure. High blood pressure increases the amount of force against artery walls. Over time, this damages the arteries, leaving them more likely to become narrowed and hardened by plaque. Injured arteries cannot deliver enough oxygen around the body. This means that high blood pressure can damage

To read more about how high blood pressure can increase your risk of heart disease, visit:

ON THE WEB

http://www.cdc.gov/dhdsp/data_statistics/fact_sheets/fs_state_hbp.htm

For more information on how to manage high blood pressure, visit:

http://www.cdc.gov/bloodpressure/what_you_can_do.htm

many tissues, including the brain (increasing the risk of stroke) and heart (increasing the risk of congestive heart failure).

If you have diabetes, your doctor will check your blood pressure at each visit to make sure it is within an acceptable range. Optimal blood pressure is considered to be less than 120/80 mm Hg, and your doctor will work with you to develop a plan to help reduce your blood pressure. This may require lifestyle changes as well as drugs:

- Eating a heart-healthy diet
- Losing weight, if this is necessary
- Exercising
- Stopping smoking if you are a smoker
- Cutting back on alcohol
- Drugs to control your high blood pressure

74. Should I take aspirin to reduce my risk of heart disease?

Aspirin can be helpful in some circumstances to reduce the risk of heart attack, some strokes, and other problems with blood flow in people who have cardiovascular disease or in those who have already suffered a heart attack or stroke. If you are one of these people, taking aspirin each day may be helpful for you.

For more information on diabetes and heart disease, see Document 15.2.Asp

ON THE DVD

For more information on how aspirin can help lower your risk of heart disease and stroke, see Document 15.2.Asp

http://www.fda.gov/downloads/Drugs/EmergencyPreparedness/Bioterrorismand DrugPreparedness/UCM133432.pdf

But as with all drugs, there are risks as well as benefits when taking aspirin, especially if you take it daily. Long-term aspirin use can lead to serious side effects, such as stomach bleeding, kidney failure, bleeding in the brain, and certain types of strokes.

So do not take aspirin daily without discussing this with your doctor. He or she will help you figure out whether taking daily aspirin each day over the long-term caries more benefits than risks for you.

75. How do different foods affect the risk of heart disease?

Diet plays a key role in the development and prevention of heart disease. A healthy diet is one that is low in sugar, salt, and saturated fats, and contains a balance of:

- Protein: choose low-fat options, such as lean meats, fish, skim milk, or other foods with high levels of protein, like legumes.
- Carbohydrates: foods high in fiber, like whole-wheat bread, fruits, vegetables, and oatmeal, are better than starchy foods like pasta or bread—especially if you have diabetes.
- Unsaturated fat: The majority of fats in your diet should be monounsaturated or polyunsaturated for heart health. Lowering your saturated fat intake helps to lower your risk of heart disease. The American Heart Association recommends making sure saturated fats in your diet do not total more than 5% to 6% of total calories (about 111 to 13 grams for someone eating 2,000 calories per day in their diet).

Make an appointment with a registered dietitian to get help making a balanced diet plan that is appropriate for your dietary needs.

76. I've had a heart attack. What happens now?

Once you have had a heart attack, a major goal will be to prevent any more from happening.

Heart disease can get worse if you do not take steps to get your heart as healthy as possible. Lifestyle plays a big role in this, so now is the time to be honest with yourself and start making whatever healthy changes you know are necessary to protect your heart.

Some changes you can make if they apply to you:

- Eat a heart-healthy diet
- Maintain a healthy weight
- Keep your blood pressure under control
- Keep your cholesterol levels under control
- Keep your blood sugar levels under control
- Exercise

- Stop smoking
- Take all your medicines properly
- Speak to your doctor about whether daily aspirin will be useful for you
- Manage the stress in your life

You can dramatically lower your risk of having another heart attack and future heart problems by making these changes. It's never too late to take steps to prevent another heart attack.

To read more about how to cope after a heart attack, visit:

http://www.nhlbi.nih.gov/health/health-topics/topics/heartattack/lifeafter.html

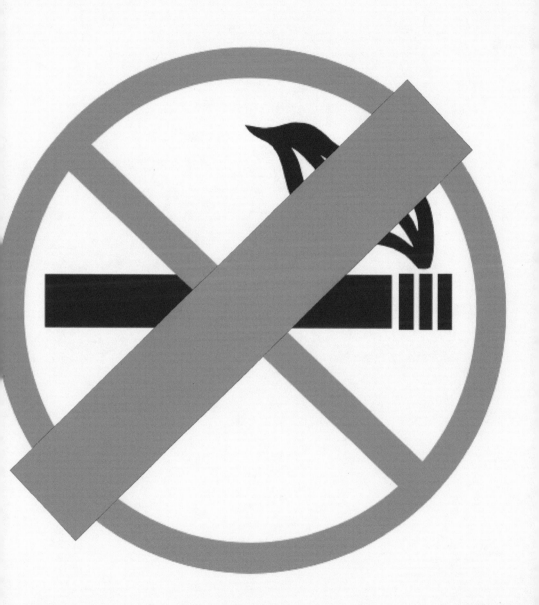

PART SIX

Keys to Living with Diabetes

In Part Six, we will discuss some important aspects of living with diabetes. We will take a look at why you should stop smoking, discussing the benefits of stopping, and some strategies to help get you started as you quit. We will also address diet, nutrition, and the management of obesity in the course of diabetes. Finally, we will answer questions on exercise, including how much exercise you need, what types are best for you, and how to get started if you have never exercised before.

CHAPTER 16
Stopping Smoking

CHAPTER 17
Diet, Nutrition, and Management of Obesity

CHAPTER 18
Physical Activity

Stopping Smoking

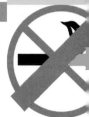

77. Why should I stop smoking?

Aside from the general reasons that you should stop smoking for the benefit of improved general health, it is especially important for people with diabetes to stop smoking, because it:

- Makes it harder to control your blood sugar levels: If you have diabetes and you smoke, it will raise your HbA1c levels.
- Affects how insulin works in your body: when you smoke, it makes your body less able to respond to insulin, and this in turn raises your blood sugar levels.
- It increases your chances of getting complications from your diabetes: these include eye problems, nerve problems, and kidney problems.
- It also increases the risk of getting heart and blood vessel problems: this can lead to heart attack, stroke, and hardening of the arteries. When problems with blood vessels lead to poor blood flow in the legs and feet, infections, ulcers, and even the need for amputation, can result.

Your risk of getting these complications increases the more you smoke, and the longer you smoke.

Also, even if you don't yet have diabetes, smoking can increase your risk of getting type 2 diabetes—research has shown that smokers are about 30% to 40% more likely to develop this disease than nonsmokers.

To learn more about the risks of smoking, and the benefits of stopping, visit:

http://www.cancer.gov/cancertopics/factsheet/Tobacco/cessation

and http://www.cdc.gov/tobacco/campaign/tips/diseases/diabetes.html

78. Why is it so hard to stop smoking?

The nicotine in tobacco is what makes it hard for people to stop smoking. It is a drug, and can be addictive because it stimulates pleasure centers in the brain and also relaxes the body. Because it is inhaled, it reaches the brain in less than ten seconds—twice as quickly as intravenous drugs, and three times faster than alcohol. Over time, smokers need more and more nicotine to get the same feeling they used to get from smaller amounts—this is because the body becomes tolerant to nicotine.

People who smoke also become physically addicted to the nicotine, because when they try to stop smoking, they suffer withdrawal symptoms—when their body doesn't get nicotine, they feel uncomfortable and crave cigarettes.

So, when smokers try to stop smoking, they have to deal with the problems of physical as well as psychological dependence. This combination makes it especially hard to give up smoking. Over time, the nicotine changes a smoker's brain chemistry, leading to strong urges to smoke. This is because every puff of smoke sends nicotine to the part of your brain that is responsible for making us do things, and therefore causes an association between the nicotine and the action. The nicotine has therefore trained this part of their brain to have a cigarette in certain psychological trigger situations—this might be immediately after a meal, or when drinking alcohol with friends, for instance.

Nicotine is the most common type of chemical addiction in the United States, and scientific research has suggested that is as addictive as alcohol, cocaine, or heroin.

NOTE

When a smoker finishes a cigarette, the nicotine level in their body starts to drop. As it gets lower and lower, the pleasant feelings from the nicotine effect wear off. This leaves the person wanting to smoke again. If there is a delay before the smoker gets another cigarette, he or she may begin to feel irritated and edgy, until they smoke the next cigarette. The uncomfortable feelings then start to wear off, and the whole cycle continues.

79. What are some strategies that might give me the best chance of stopping?

About 95% of people who try to stop smoking tend to relapse within one year, with about half of them relapsing within the first week. A large number of these people try to go it alone, however, and it is extremely hard to stop smoking without any help.

Planning ahead can therefore be helpful. So, when you decide to stop smoking, acknowledge why you are doing it—stopping smoking will lead to many beneficial effects on your health, and will help you live longer.

Stopping smoking has many health benefits.

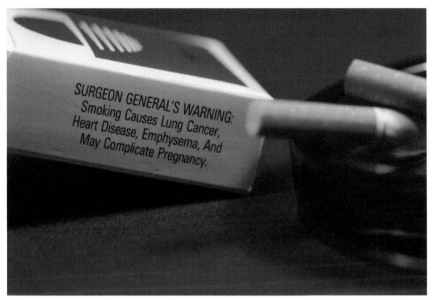

SOURCE: Wikimedia Commons.

The next step is choosing a Quit Day. Pick a date that isn't too far away, but gives you enough time to do as much planning as you need—and write the date on your calendar.

In the run-up to Quit Day

- Tell family and friends about your decision and share your Quit Day with them.
- Throw out any cigarettes and ashtrays you have at home, at work, or in the car.
- Collect some "substitutes," like sugar-free gum, candy, or even things like toothpicks that you can hold in your hand and put in your mouth instead of a cigarette if you need to.
- Practice saying, "No thanks, I don't smoke."
- Decide what your support system will be. If you prefer to use a support group, start searching for one in your area. Or if you are choosing to use your family and friends for support, get advice from those who have been successful at quitting smoking, and ask those who still smoke to avoid smoking around you.

- If you would like to use medicines, speak to your doctor well in advance, so that you have everything you need in time for your Quit Day.

On your Quit Day

- Keep busy! Go to the gym, or get out for a run or a walk—whatever you can do to keep your mind off the desire to smoke.
- Stay away from other smokers.
- Avoid situations that might trigger you wanting to smoke.
- Avoid drinking alcohol.
- Attend a support group meeting if there is one locally.
- If you have decided on **nicotine replacement therapy (NRT)**, start taking it. Using NRT or prescription medicines is considered to double your chance of quitting smoking, and can help with withdrawal symptoms and nicotine cravings.
- Most importantly, don't smoke!

For more information on strategies to help you stop smoking, see Document 16.1.Stop

http://circ.ahajournals.org/content/104/11/e51.full.pdf+html

For information on some different medicines available to help you stop smoking, see Document 16.2.Meds

http://www.fda.gov/downloads/ForConsumers/ByAudience/ForWomen/FreePublications/UCM364679.pdf

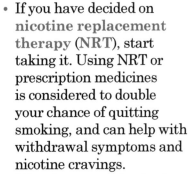

For additional strategies to help you stop smoking, visit:

http://www.nhlbi.nih.gov/health/health-topics/topics/smo/strategies.html

Nevertheless, millions of Americans have managed to stop smoking, so despite the difficulty, it can be done. Many experts believe that one key to success is having plenty of face-to-face encouragement from friends, family members, and doctors along the way.

80. I've heard about "withdrawal"—what should I expect?

Withdrawal symptoms are the physical sensations that occur when a smoker tries to stop smoking. They happen because the body has become physically addicted to the nicotine, and needs it to feel good. This can happen after even a few weeks of smoking. When a smoker tries to stop smoking and is no longer getting nicotine, the body goes into nicotine withdrawal. The symptoms of withdrawal are many and varied, and can include:

- Dizziness
- Headaches
- Irritability
- Restlessness
- Difficulty concentrating
- Problems sleeping
- Anxiety
- Depression
- Increased appetite

It takes a little time to get over the withdrawal symptoms. Although many of the physical feelings disappear after a few days of not smoking, the cravings take longer to go away.

ON THE WEB

For information on how to handle withdrawal and cravings, visit:

http://smokefree.gov/withdrawal

and http://smokefree.gov/cravings

81. What if I slip-up and smoke again?

If you slip-up while trying to stop smoking, don't despair. A survey by the American Lung Association found that 6 out of 10 former smokers did not stop smoking successfully on their first try, and required multiple attempts to quit for good.

Slip-up

If it was a true slip-up, this is a one-time event that can be corrected immediately—just continue to not smoke as if nothing happened.

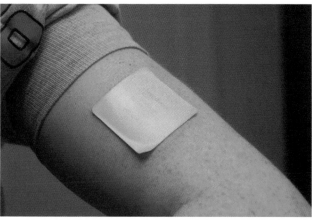

◀ FIGURE 16.2
Nicotine replacement therapy in the form of a nicotine patch.

SOURCE: Wikimedia Commons.

Relapse

If, however, you relapsed back into smoking, you still shouldn't despair—just set a new Quit Day, and get started again. Think about you previous attempts to stop smoking—make a list of what worked well for you, and what didn't. And think about what you can do differently this time:

- If you didn't previously join a support group, find one locally and give it a try.
- If you didn't use NRT or any other medicines to help you quit smoking, speak to your doctor about trying one (see Figure 16.2).
- Get advice from friends and family members who have ultimately been successful, but had slip-ups or relapses on the way.

For more encouragement on how to deal with slip-ups while you are trying to stop smoking, visit:

ON THE WEB

http://smokefree.gov/slips

Nicotine withdrawal is one of the toughest challenges you will experience. So be sure to stay positive, and take things one day at a time. Use any slip-ups as learning experiences, not excuses to go back to smoking.

82. How soon will I begin to see the health benefits of not smoking?

The benefits of stopping smoking are huge, and your body will begin to experience them immediately:

First 24 hours

- Heart rate decreases within just 20 minutes
- Breathing will be easier
- The level of carbon monoxide in your blood drops to normal

Within 2 months

- Circulation improves
- Lung function improves
- Skin condition improves
- Bad breath improves

Within 6 months to a year

- Heartburn improves
- Risk of coronary heart disease is reduced to half that of someone who continues to smoke
- Coughing and phlegm production disappear

Within 5 to 15 years

- The risk of cancer of the mouth, throat, esophagus, and bladder is halved
- The risk of certain diseases is reduced or eliminated. For instance, the risk of stroke drops to the same level as that of a nonsmoker by 2 to 5 years.
- By 10 years, the risk of dying from lung cancer is about half that of someone who continues to smoke
- By 15 years, the risk of coronary heart disease is similar to that of a nonsmoker

For every day you keep smoking after about your mid-thirties, you lose around 6 hours of life. It has been estimated that smokers live an 18-hour day until they stop smoking. The good news, however, is that immediately when you stop smoking, you begin to get back your life expectancy at a rate of 6 hours per day.

It's never too late to stop smoking— no matter how old you are, there will always be some benefit from stopping, and from stopping as soon as you can. Even if it takes multiple tries to stop, the eventual benefits are far greater than the negative side of smoking.

To see a video discussing how quickly your body experiences benefits after you stop smoking, visit:

http://www.youtube.com/watch?v=SlKqiJ3Coqw

83. Will I gain weight when I stop smoking?

Although many smokers gain weight when they quit smoking, not all do. Even in those who do, studies have shown that most people gain just 4 to 10 pounds. A good way to help reduce any weight gain when you stop smoking, is to increase your exercise level.

To learn about some ways to help control your weight while you stop smoking, visit WIN, the Weight-control Information Network:

ON THE WEB

http://www.win.niddk.nih.gov/

Many people don't stop smoking because they do not want to gain weight. The weight gain is usually small, and this is less harmful to the body than continuing to smoke. The best advice is to conquer the nicotine addiction first, and then tackle any weight gain later on.

CHAPTER
17 *Diet, Nutrition, and Management of Obesity*

84. How does diet affect blood sugar control?

Food contains three food groups: carbohydrates, protein, and fat. All are required for optimal health, but they have different effects on your blood sugar levels after eating. It is important to understand how these different food groups affect your blood sugar levels—this is one of the main steps toward making healthier food choices.

Carbohydrates

Carbohydrates are present in starchy foods like pasta, cereal, bread, and rice, as well as in milk, fruit, vegetables, and sweet things. Foods that are high in carbohydrates will have the biggest effect on your blood sugar levels. Eating large amounts of foods containing carbohydrates will lead to higher blood sugar levels after a meal.

Protein

Protein is found in animal products, like meat, fish, and dairy products, as well as in things like beans and nuts. Protein does not affect your blood sugar level very much.

Fat

There are four main types of fats:

- **monounsaturated fats** (good fats—found in olive oil, olives, nuts)
- **polyunsaturated fats** (good fats—found in salmon, tuna, tofu, soybean oil)

- trans fats (bad fats—found in butter, cheese, ice cream, high-fat cuts of meat)
- saturated fats (bad fats—found in candy bars, stick margarine, packaged snack foods, fried foods)

Foods containing fat will slow down how quickly the stomach empties after a meal. This can result in lower blood sugar levels just after a meal, and higher levels later on after a meal.

85. How much should I be eating?

The number of calories you eat each day has the biggest effect on your body weight. So it is important to regulate your total daily calorie intake, especially if you have diabetes and need to lose weight. The number of calories you should eat each day is based on your very individual needs. However, as an approximate guide, each day you should eat:

- **1,200 to 1,600 calories**: if you are a small woman who exercises; a medium-sized woman who doesn't exercise a lot; a small- to medium-sized woman who wants to lose some weight.
- **1,600 to 2,000 calories**: if you are a large-sized man or woman who wants to lose some weight; a small man at a healthy weight; or a medium-sized man who does not exercise a lot.
- **2,000 to 2,400 calories:** if you are a medium to large-sized man or woman who exercises a lot or is physically active; or a large man at a healthy weight.

ON THE WEB

For more information about calories and weight management, visit:

http://www.choosemyplate.gov/weight-management-calories/calories.html

You should work with your doctor or a registered dietitian to determine how many calories you need for your age, sex, and activity level, in particular.

The newest food model, MyPlate, released by the U.S. Department of Agriculture (USDA) is based on a nutrition counseling method called the "plate method." This is used to counsel people on how to eat if they have diabetes, as well as just for a general healthy diet. It is a simple method that only involves using an image of a plate divided into different sections that contain different types of foods—this simple visual lets you picture a balanced meal plan

▼ **FIGURE 17.1**
The My Plate food model.

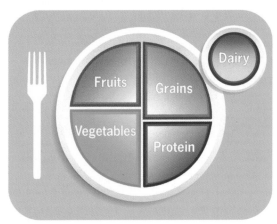

SOURCE: Shutterstock.

on a plate. No special tools are needed to figure out how you are supposed to eat—it simply involves eating less meats and starchy foods, while filling your plate with more non-starchy vegetables. Eating less starchy carbohydrates will not only help to lower your blood sugar levels after a meal, but will also help you lose excess weight.

For more information on how much to eat, and what types of foods to eat, visit:

ON THE WEB

http://www.diabetes.niddk.nih.gov/dm/pubs/eating_ez/#pyramid

and http://diabetes.about.com/gi/o.htm?zi=1/XJ&zTi=1&sdn=diabetes&cdn=health&tm=1021&f=00&su=p284.13.342.p_&tt=2&bt=3&bts=3&zu=http%3A//www.choosemyplate.gov/

Visit a registered dietitian for advice on how much you should be eating each day, and particularly how much carbohydrate you should have at each meal. He or she can also advise you on how to measure or estimate portions at home.

86. What kind of diet do I need to follow?

The American Diabetes Association (ADA) does not recommend any one specific type of diet for people with diabetes. Instead, their position is that an eating plan should be very individual, and based on the person's needs, as well as cultural and lifestyle factors. In research trials, no specific type of diet has proven to be better than another for people with diabetes. Some benefit has been shown in some people who followed a low carbohydrate diet, while others had benefit from a high protein, vegan diet. So it is important to speak to a registered dietitian for guidance on what is the right type of meal plan for you if you have diabetes or pre-diabetes.

Some people often refer to the ABCs of a diabetes diet, meaning that a person with diabetes should eat in such a way that pays particular attention to these three things:

1. A is for HbA1c

2. B is for blood pressure

3. C is for cholesterol

For best control of diabetes and to reduce the risk of its complications, these things need to be well controlled and as close to normal as possible.

Regardless of the meal plan you come up with to manage your diabetes, a heart-healthy approach is a good one to take (see questions 72 and 75 for more information), and will certainly target the ABCs of diabetes.

87. What foods should I avoid eating?

Making healthy food choices is the key to managing your diabetes, and in many cases, moderation is the key. But although having diabetes doesn't mean you have to deprive yourself, there are certainly some foods that you are best to avoid or limit. These include:

- Candy
- Fried foods
- Fast food
- High-carbohydrate baked goods
- Foods or drinks with added sugar
- Processed lunch meats
- Restaurant hamburgers
- Frozen meals
- Regular soft drinks
- Processed snack food
- Alcohol

Many of these foods are either loaded with sugar, fat, or calories, or have high sodium levels, and are best avoided even by people without diabetes.

88. What do I need to know about carbohydrates?

Although carbohydrates affect your blood sugar control more than proteins and fats, you still need them in your diet. So you need help from your doctor and a registered dietitian to find a balance of carbohydrates in your diet that is healthy for you, and will keep your risk of diabetes complications as low as possible.

When you have determined how much carbohydrate is appropriate for your diet, you can begin to use the "carbohydrate counting" technique as you plan your meals. This will help you manage your blood sugar levels and keep them in the target range that your doctor has determined is best for you.

How much carbohydrate you eat will be based on your personal needs, such as your age, level of activity, and what medicines you take, although, according to the American Diabetes Association, 45 to 60 grams is a good starting point to consider for each meal.

How much carbohydrate is in foods?

Food labels on packaged products tell you how much carbohydrate is in each item, so you should read the label if one is present—look at the number of grams of total carbohydrate, and pay close attention to the serving size that contains this amount of carbohydrate. Knowing how much carbohydrate you can eat at each meal, you can calculate what portion size you can have.

For foods that are not packaged, and don't have a label, you will need to learn to estimate how much carbohydrate they contain. For example, the following food servings contain about 15 grams of carbohydrate:

For information on carbohydrate counting, visit:

http://diabetes.niddk.nih.gov/dm/pubs/carbohydrate_ez/index.aspx

http://www.nlm.nih.gov/medlineplus/ency/patientinstructions/000321.htm

ON THE WEB

- 1 slice of bread
- ½ a cup of casserole
- ½ cup of black beans
- ¼ of a large (3 oz) baked potato
- 4 to 6 crackers
- 2 small cookies

89. What are the "glycemic index" and "glycemic load"?

Both of these terms are related, but represent different concepts:

Glycemic index (GI) is a way of measuring how much a food affects blood sugar. Based on this, foods are given a GI score from 0 and 100.

Low GI (Score 55 or lower)

Foods with a low GI include things like:

- Skim milk
- Oatmeal
- Kidney beans
- Carrots
- Most fruits (except watermelon and those listed in the medium GI group)

Foods with a low GI usually make blood sugar levels lower than those in the other two groups.

Medium GI (Score 56 to 69)

Foods with a medium GI include things like:

- Grapes
- Bananas
- Corn-on-the-cob
- Ice cream

Foods with a medium GI usually lead to blood sugar levels in between those due to foods in the low and high GI food list.

High GI (Score 70 or higher)

Foods with a high GI include things like:

- Baked goods
- Pasta
- Rice
- White bread

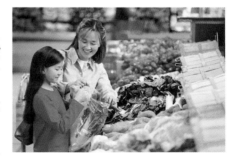

Foods with a high GI usually make blood sugar levels higher. People who eat a lot of food with a high GI typically have more body fat when measured by their body mass index (BMI).

The glycemic load (GL) is a measure of how much carbohydrate is in a food, and therefore how much it will affect your blood sugar level after you have eaten it. It is similar to GI, but also takes serving size into account, and therefore represents a practical way of applying the GI score in your meal planning.

To calculate GL, you take the number of grams in the serving of carbohydrate, multiply it by the GI, and then divide the answer by 100. In theory, a food with a GL of one point will raise blood sugar levels as much as one gram of sugar would.

Diets with a low GL will have a low GI. Some of the effects of foods with a low GL include:

- Keeping blood sugar levels more stable
- Burning more calories
- Making weight loss easier

Therefore they are considered to be more heart-healthy.

Low GL (Score 10 or lower)

- Whole-wheat breads
- High-fiber fruits and vegetables like apples, watermelon, green peas, and carrots
- Milk
- Cereals made with 100% bran
- Lentils

Medium GL (Score 11 to 19)

- Whole-wheat pasta
- Oatmeal
- Sweet potato
- Brown rice
- Fruit juices without added sugar

High GL (Score 20 or higher)

- Candy
- Sweetened fruit juices
- High-sugar drinks
- White pasta
- White rice
- Pizza

To read more about GI and GL, visit:

http://newsinhealth.nih.gov/ issue/dec2012/feature2

ON THE WEB

Considering the GL of foods can be an important way for people with diabetes to help manage their blood sugar levels and keep them stable.

If you are obese and having problems losing weight through lifestyle changes like diet and exercise, prescription medicines may be an option to help you. They are not a substitute for a healthy lifestyle, but when combined with diet and exercise, can help people lose up to 10% of their body weight.

Three of the prescription medicines are approved for long-term use, and are taken for several months at a time:

- **Orlistat**: Stops some of the fat in your diet from being taken up by the body.
- **Lorcaserin**: Works on chemical receptors in the brain, so you eat less and may feel full after eating smaller meals.
- **Phentermine-topiramate**: A combination of phentermine (to reduce appetite) and topiramate (usually used as an anti-seizure medication, but one of its side effects is weight loss).

Other appetite suppressing drugs are also available that are only approved for use for a shorter length of time (up to 12 weeks). These are:

- Phentermine (the most commonly used of this group of appetite suppressants)
- Benzphetamine
- Diethylpropion
- Phendimetrazine

These cause weight loss by stimulating brain chemicals to make a person feel full sooner, or less hungry.

Sometimes doctors use other drugs "off label" to help people lose weight. This means that they are licensed for use for a different health problem, but have proven helpful in causing weight loss in some people. One example of this is metformin, a drug used for treatment of type 2 diabetes.

For more information on some prescription drugs used to treat obesity, along with their benefits and side effects, see Document 17.1.Obes

http://win.niddk.nih.gov/publications/PDFs/Prescriptionmeds1104bw.pdf

Bariatric surgery is also known as weight loss surgery. It is the term given to the various operations that are carried out on people who are obese. It is often used on patients who have severe obesity who are having difficulty losing weight by means of diet, physical exercise, and weight loss medicines.

The aim of bariatric surgery is to carry out a procedure that will reduce how much food the patient can eat. It also interferes with digestion, so food is not broken down and absorbed as usual—it reduces how much food is absorbed by the stomach and intestines after a meal.

Most bariatric surgery is now carried out by laparoscopy, instead of open surgery which involves opening up the abdomen. This is less damaging to the body tissues, and allows for quicker healing and fewer postoperative complications.

Types of operations

There are four types of bariatric surgery used:

- Adjustable gastric band
- Roux-en-Y gastric bypass
- Biliopancreatic diversion with a duodenal switch
- Vertical sleeve gastrectomy

▼ FIGURE 17.2
Roux-en-Y gastric bypass procedure.

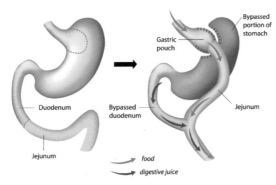

SOURCE: Shutterstock

The Roux-en-Y gastric bypass technique is the most common form of weight loss surgery carried out. In this operation, the surgeon divides the stomach into a large portion and a very small portion, and then staples the small portion into a small pouch. The stomach pouch is then disconnected from the first part of the intestine (the duodenum). The stomach is then reconnected to the second part of the intestine (the jejunum).

The adjustable gastric band procedure is the second most common form. The U.S. Food and Drug Administration (FDA) approves the use of this procedure for people with a body mass index (BMI) of 30 kg/m^2 or more who also have at least one of the following conditions:

- Heart disease
- Type 2 diabetes
- Arthritis
- Severe obstructive sleep apnea

However, there are risks and complications associated with having this type of surgery. In addition to the risks due to surgery and anesthesia (such as internal bleeding, blood clots in the

The risk of dying soon after weight loss surgery is estimated at about 1 in 200.

legs that can move to the heart and lungs, and even death), patients may be left with a lot of loose skin after the operation. However, the most common side effects include vomiting, diarrhea, nausea, bloating, excessive sweating, dizziness, and increased gas.

One long-term problem after weight loss surgery, especially after gastric bypass, is the problem known as dumping syndrome. This happens in up to half of patients who undergo weight loss surgery, and is due to food moving too quickly through the intestines. When this occurs, patients may sweat and experience weakness, nausea, faintness, and diarrhea after eating. This can be prevented by avoiding high-sugar foods and eating high-fiber foods instead.

Patients also have to understand that changes will be needed after the operation. They must to ready to make changes in their lifestyle to keep the weight off. This involves sticking to a strict diet and exercise plan for the rest of their life to keep the weight off.

For more information on the types of bariatric surgery, as well as their advantages and side effects, visit:

http://win.niddk.nih.gov/publications/gastric.htm

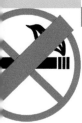

CHAPTER 18 *Physical Activity*

92. Why should I exercise?

Exercise is important for everyone because it improves overall health and fitness, helps with weight loss, and even helps you manage stress. For example, it builds muscle strength, improves blood circulation and lowers blood pressure, and reduces the risk of heart disease and stroke. It also helps protect against some cancers, and lowers your risk of major chronic diseases by up to 50%, also reducing the risk of early death by up to 30%.

And if you have diabetes, it will also help you improve your blood sugar control and reduce the amount of diabetes medicine you need.

For more information on the benefits of exercise, visit:

ON THE WEB

http://www.cdc.gov/physical activity/everyone/health/

For additional information on how much physical activity you need, visit:

ON THE WEB

http://www.cdc.gov/physicalactivity/ everyone/guidelines/index.html

and http://www.health.gov/paguidelines/ blog/post/How-Much-Daily-Exercise-is-Best-for-Weight-Loss.aspx

93. How much exercise do I need?

Experts recommend you should get at least 150 minutes of moderate exercise each week (30 minutes of exercise at least 5 days each week).

94. What kinds of physical activity are best for me?

Your doctor will be able to help you decide what types of exercise are best for you, based on your diabetes and other medical history. If you are just starting to exercise for the first time, you may be advised to start out light (see Question 95).

However, if you are not new to exercising, you should aim for 150 minutes of moderate intensity aerobic exercise each week (see Question 93). Moderate intensity exercise means that you should feel like your body is warming up, and you should break out into a little sweat. However, you should also be able to talk and have a conversation while you exercise.

Aerobic exercise activities include things such as:

- Fast walking
- Light jogging

- Bicycling
- Swimming

What if I have diabetes complications?

Be careful with exercise if you suffer from diabetes complications. If you have diabetic foot problems, for instance, your feet might be numb and you might not realize you have sores on your feet. These sores might worsen if you exercise. If you have diabetic eye problems, these can be made worse by lifting heavy weights, due to the increase in pressure in blood vessels in your eyes as you lift. So, be sure to talk to your doctor before exercising if this is the case. He or she can advise you on what types of exercise will be best for you to avoid worsening any diabetic complications you may have.

For some ideas on different types of physical activities, visit:

https://www.womenshealth.gov/fitness-nutrition/how-to-be-active-for-health/type-of-physical-activity.html

95. I've never exercised before—how do I get started?

If you are new to exercise, it is important to speak to your doctor before starting out, to make sure you are fit to start exercising, and to get advice on what types of activity might be best for you to begin with.

For ideas on how to make regular exercise a part of your day, visit:

http://www.choosemyplate.gov/physical-activity/increase-physical-activity.html

Starting an exercise regime for the first time can be very intimidating for some people, but in general, it is best to start small. You can begin with even as little as 10 minutes walking each day, and work your way up gradually, adding extra 10-minute sessions each day as your fitness level improves and you become stronger.

96. How will exercise affect my blood sugar?

Although exercise is important it does bring some challenges for people with diabetes, especially those who take insulin or other medicines that can lower blood sugar levels. So, because exercise can also affect your blood sugar, it is important to remember to check it before and after exercise—and even during your workout if it is a long or strenuous one, or if you feel weak or faint, or have any other reason to feel the need to check it. This will allow you to see whether your sugar levels are staying steady, and help you decide if it is safe to keep exercising.

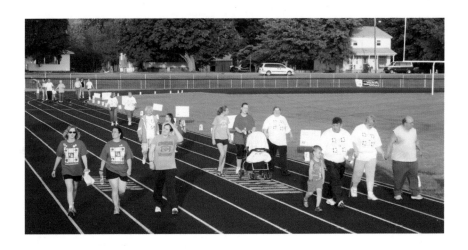

Hypoglycemia

Hypoglycemia (low blood sugar) is the biggest risk for people with diabetes when they exercise, particularly with moderate or strenuous exercise. So for this reason, avoid scheduling your workout at the same time as your insulin level is about to peak, because this will already be working to lower your blood sugar levels, and exercise will just add to this effect and lower your blood sugar even more. The same applies if you are using any other diabetes medicines that work to lower your blood sugar levels—think about the timing of your exercise in relation to when the effect of your medicine will peak.

Hyperglycemia

You should also avoid exercise if you have hyperglycemia (high blood sugar). So, if your blood sugar level is 250 mg/dL or higher, or if you have ketones in your urine, do not exercise until both levels are normal again (see Question 97).

For additional information on exercising when you have diabetes, see Document 18.1.PE

ON THE WEB

http://diabetes.niddk.nih.gov/dm/pubs/
physical_ez/physactivity_508.pdf

Careful monitoring of your blood sugar is the most essential strategy to help keep your blood sugar levels steady while you exercise. Don't wait for your body to show symptoms of low blood sugar—it is important for you to be in charge of doing everything to prevent this from happening while you exercise.

When to check your blood sugar levels

You should check your blood sugar levels:

- 30 minutes before exercising: in general, your blood sugar should be between 100 and 250 mg/dL for exercise.
  - If it is lower than 100 mg/dL, eat at least 15 to 20 grams of fast-acting carbohydrate (such as a regular soda, or some glucose tablets) before your workout.
  - If it is higher than 250 mg/dL, you should test your urine for ketones. If it is positive for ketones, do not exercise until they are no longer present, or are at a low level.
  - If it is higher than 300 mg/dL, you are at increased risk of dehydration and diabetic ketoacidosis. Test your urine for ketones. Do not exercise until the sugar level drops to normal again, and your urine contains no ketones, or they are at a low level.
- Every 30 minutes during your exercise regime.
- 30 minutes after you finish exercising.

What do I do about hypoglycemia?

Be very mindful of symptoms of hypoglycemia during your workout. Stop exercising immediately if you feel dizzy, weak, shaky, confused, or faint. If you check your blood sugar during or after exercise, and discover that you are hypoglycemic, you should treat it just the same way as you would treat it at any other time.

- Have at least 15 to 20 grams of fast-acting carbohydrate (such as a regular soda, or some glucose tablets)
- Rest for 15 minutes and recheck your blood sugar

- Repeat the carbohydrate treatment if your blood sugar is still low or you have symptoms of hypoglycemia
- Rest for another 15 minutes and recheck you blood sugar

Repeat these steps until your blood sugar returns to normal. If you would like to go back to exercising, make sure your blood sugar level is above 100 mg/dL before doing so.

If you have any concerns about your symptoms, or if your blood sugar level is not returning to normal, do not return to exercising, and seek medical help immediately.

What else can I do to be prepared for changes in blood sugar when I exercise?

- Take a carbohydrate source with you
- Take a blood sugar monitor with you
- Exercise in public places, in case you need help
- Take a cellphone with you
- Be sure to carry your medical ID with you

What about after I exercise

Your body can experience improvement in blood sugar levels for up to 3 days after you finish exercising. So be sure to keep a check on your blood sugar during this time, because it may be lower than usual, and you may need to adjust your diabetes medicines to match this change.

▶ **FIGURE 18.1**
Monitoring blood sugar levels is important when you exercise.

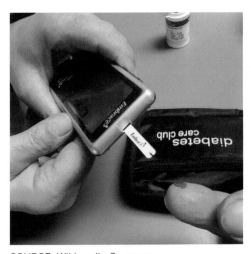

SOURCE: Wikimedia Commons

Index

Pills, control blood sugar, 54
Pioglitazone, 55
Polyunsaturated fats, 112
Pre-eclampsia, 72
Pre-mixed insulin, 62
Prediabetes, 4, 41
Pregnancy, 71–72
    hormones and gestational
        diabetes., 75
Protein, 101, 112

R

Renin inhibitors, 69
Repaglinide, 56
Retinopathy. *See* Diabetic eye
    disease

S

Saturated fats, 113
Secondary diabetes, 26
Sexual problems, diabetes,
    95–96
Sitagliptin, 56
Smoking, 103–112
Somatostatin, 10
Statins, 27
Stroke, 4
Sugar, levels of, 3
Sulfonylureas, 55

T

Thiazide diuretics, 27
Thirst, excessive, 33, 34
Tiredness, unusual, 33, 34
Trans fats, 113
Triglycerides, 70
Trypsin, 9
Type 1 diabetes
    causes, 16–18
    risk for, 18–19
    symptoms of, 33–34
Type 2 diabetes, 4
    causes, 20–21
    risk for, 21–23
    symptoms of, 34–37

U

Unsaturated fat, 101
Urination, 33

V

Vision, blurred, 34

W

Weight gain, 34
Weight loss, 33, 34
Weight loss surgery, 6. *See also*
    Bariatric surgery
Withdrawal symptoms, 108